The
Dictionary of
Medical Folklore

The Dictionary of Medical Folklore

CAROL ANN RINZLER

THOMAS Y. CROWELL, PUBLISHERS
Established 1834 / New York

FIRST EDITION

Designed by C. Linda Dingler

Library of Congress Cataloging in Publication Data

Rinzler, Carol Ann.
  Dictionary of medical folklore.
  Includes index.
  1. Folk medicine. 2. Medicine, Popular. 3. Medical
delusions. I. Title.
GR880.R53 1979   615'.882   78–69518
ISBN 0–690–01704–9

79 80 81 82 83 10 9 8 7 6 5 4 3 2 1

31617

For my husband

Introduction

No matter how sophisticated we grow, most of us still believe, however surreptitiously, in magic, and most of the magic we believe has to do with medicine.

Is there a place anywhere on earth where people have grown up without a literature of magical medical advice? I doubt it. We may call these bits and pieces of advice old wives' tales and publicly sneer at their naïveté, but who among us is absolutely certain, one hundred percent, that an apple a day does *not* keep the doctor away or that we cannot avoid colds simply by keeping our feet dry?

Now, like most writers, I am an inveterate collector of newspaper and magazine clippings. At home, in the doctor's office, in someone else's living room—the magazines I've already read are easy to spot. They're the ones with the slightly moth-eaten look.

My passion for clipping, though, is not matched by an equal passion for filing. I really envy writers who keep their clippings neatly filed. I once read that Theodore White (or was it Arthur Schlesinger?) actually travels with an expandable alphabetized folder, so that things are in order right from the start. That's my idea of real class, but it's not the way I do it.

The way I do it is this: I toss all my clippings into a large manila envelope on the back of my desk and, every other month or so, when the envelope is full enough so that it is tipping over, I sort through the clippings to see if anything important has floated to the top.

Because I am most interested in medical subjects, virtually all the things I clip are about medicine. About four years ago, during one bimonthly sorting session, I noticed that I had an interesting little collection of clippings about medical old wives' tales. Some of the clippings seemed to prove one tale or another true; some of them, false; and some were somewhere in the middle.

Clearly, however, there was something incubating in the clippings, and the first tangible result was an article on fifty of the more common old wives' tales, which ran in *Glamour* in April, 1975. After that, I sort of assumed that the collection of medical myths would simply end up decently buried in the file drawer I keep for completed articles. But, to my surprise, the pile of clippings kept growing. Day after day, I came across nifty snippets in the newspapers, the magazines, and the books I read. By the middle of 1977, I had four manila envelopes full of medical myths tipping over on the back of the desk. Almost in self-defense—I certainly couldn't throw them out, and if I didn't bring some order to them, they would probably have spread clear across the room—I started to write this book.

By the time I finished the last page of the manuscript, which, as with my original sources, I'd assembled in assorted bits and odd-sized pieces, there were more than five hundred entries on my list. Actually, to be maddeningly accurate about it, I counted 534. I'm sure we've gained or lost a few in the editing. Nevertheless—would you believe it?—as soon as the book was set in type and couldn't be changed anymore, that folder of clippings on my desk began to fill up again.

So I have no doubt at all that despite the 534 or 535 or 536 entries in this book, one of your favorites is bound to be missing. If so, please drop me a note, in care of my publisher (Thomas Y. Crowell, 10 East 53 Street, New York, New York 10022). If I can, I'll track down the truth or falsity of your own piece of folklore on the chance that it can be put into a later edition of the Dictionary.

The same goes for any up-to-the-minute changes in scientific evaluation or any advances in research that validate or disprove one of the medical old wives' tales. Nothing is more frustrating than picking up the newspaper on the morning after the book is done to find that some researcher in some laboratory somewhere in the world has just come up with something that wipes out whole paragraphs you've written. Once again, the only remedy is rewriting in a later edition.

While I haven't put specific references in the text, I do think you might be interested in seeing a list of the sources from which I collected my material. Sometimes, it's noted right in the entry. Otherwise, my sources include the following array of journals, magazines, newspapers, textbooks, dictionaries and books on various ordinary and esoteric subjects, all listed in no particular order except one that appears logical to me.

First on the list is the marvelous *Merck Index,* the dictionary of chemicals and their origins that often gives surprising clues as to why one natural substance or another has real medical value. Then there are the standards: *The Journal of the American Medical Association, Lancet, Science, Science News,* and the more popular version, *Science Digest.* The daily newspapers (the New York *Times,* the New York *News,* the New York *Post*) and their medical columnists, including Jane Brody, Dr. Jean Mayer and Johanna Dwyer and Dr. Neil Solomon, provide a virtual treasure trove. In addition, a lively public interest in things medical makes it inevitable that there are always a few little gems tucked away in the health and/or beauty columns of such diverse publications as *Cosmopolitan, Glamour, Harper's Bazaar, Viva, Playboy* and *Penthouse,* not to mention *Consumer Reports, Newsweek, Reader's Digest,* and *Time.*

Then there are the books. Among those which yielded up fascinating snippets are *Totally Natural Beauty* by Nona Aguilar; *Fat and Thin* by Anne Scott Beller; *The Dictionary of Misinformation* by Tom Burnam; *Bizarre Plants* by William Emboden; *How Long Will I Live?* by Lawrence Galton; *Ask the Doctor* by Morris Fishbein; *Headaches* by Arthur Freese; *The People's Pharmacy* by Joe Graedon; *Blood* by Earle Hackett; *The Book of Garlic* by Lloyd Harris; *The Taste of America* by John and Karen Hess; *The Consumer's Guide to Successful Surgery* by Seymour Isenberg and L.N. Elting;

Eater's Digest by Michael Jacobsen; *Doctor!* by G. Timothy Johnson, M.D.; *Folk Medicine* by Francis Kennell; *Other Healers, Other Cures* by Helen Kroger; *Natural Foods and Nutrition Handbook* by Raphael Macia; *Hazards of Medication* by Eric Martin, *et al.; Journey* by Robert and Suzanne Massie; *Symptoms,* edited by Sigmund Stephen Miller; *Our Bodies, Ourselves* from the Boston Women's Health Book Collective; *Body Weather* by Bruce Palmer; *The Neutral Spirit* and *The Orange Man* by Berton Roueché; *The Body* by Anthony Smith; *New Wives' Tales* by Lendon H. Smith; *Simon's Book of World Sex Records* by G. L. Simon; *The Truth about Weight Control* by Neil Solomon; *Grannies' Remedies* by Mai Thomas; *Panic in the Pantry* by Elizabeth Whalen and Frederick Stare; and *Super Skin* by Jonathan Zizmor and John Foreman.

Do all those books and magazines seem a rather bloodless way to do research? If so, then I really must hasten to add that there were a lot of perfectly delightful people who took time away from their own work days to answer questions for me and sometimes, caught up in the fascination of the medical mythology, to offer some entries of their own. One woman at the Brooklyn Botanic Garden, for example, spent a few minutes talking about the effects (or non-effects) of mushrooms on silver spoons and then threw in an old wives' tale about plants left in bedrooms overnight.

In addition, the Environmental Protection Agency spokespeople steered me to sources on radiation, the people at the Hemophilia Foundation and the Genetic Counseling Services in New York helped me unravel my sentences on genetic and hereditary diseases. I found the same helpful attitudes at the Mount Sinai Medical Center in New York, the National Weather Service and the Office of the Chief Medical Examiner of the City of New York. I am a great believer in just picking up the phone and asking questions of whoever answers and I must say I was never disappointed.

And then there were The Doctors, which is how I think of the group of men and women to whom I have become accustomed to turnng for medical and dental information. Over the years, I have pestered them without mercy for solutions to various physiological puzzles and Stanley Darrow, Philip Henneman, Milton Ingerman,

David Krohn, Edith Langner, Sanford Langsam, Louis Linn, Julius N. Obin, Martin Portnoy, Sidney Rothstein and Seymour Schutzer have always responded with good-humored good grace. Naturally, their information was always impeccable; any errors in interpretation are mine.

I appreciate, too, the help of Stanley and Gladys Edelman, Helen Hand, Jean Luntz, Arline Harris, Andrea Rosen, Jackie Snyder-Luntz, Dodie Schultz and Dr. Marvin Speck, not to mention my grandparents, parents, sister, aunts, uncles and cousins, each of whom knows exactly which entry he or she tacked on to the list.

Finally, some words of pure gratitude for the people who put it all together. Cynthia Vartan, who liked the idea in the first place; Arnold Dolin, the editor who saw it through to the last page; and copyeditor Carol E.W. Edwards who, as copyeditors somehow always manage to do, got every word in the right place. Spelled right, too.

July 1978   CAROL ANN RINZLER

A

✳

---

acne.

     Acne is an adolescent problem. Most cases of acne do start during adolescence. In fact, according to figures from the National Center for Health Statistics, three out of every four American teenagers have acne to some degree. Some doctors have said that up to 80 percent of the people who first get acne as teenagers can expect to see an occasional spot or two or three well into their twenties, thirties, and sometimes forties.

    In some cases, though, the acne doesn't even begin until the thirties. Adult acne seems to hit women more often than men. (During adolescence, the rate is nearly equal: 66.4 out of every 100 boys and 69.38 out of every 100 girls have some acne at some time.) It shows up usually around the time of the menstrual period and may flare up in relation to The Pill, both when the woman is using it and when she goes off it.

     Sunbathing cures acne. Taken in moderation, exposure to the sun may help dry up superficial eruptions. However, if you exercise strenuously in the sun, or get a severe sunburn, you will stimulate the production of perspiration and/or oil, and the inevitable results will be more clogged pores and thus more infections.

Acne is caused by bacteria. The basic acne bumps and lumps are the result of hormonal action or imbalance in your own body. However, if you poke at them, these bumps can become infected by the bacteria on your face or by the bacteria you leave there from your fingertips.

Acne is contagious. No, but if the original lumps become infected the secondary bacterial infection can be passed from one person to another. You can even spread it around on your own face or body.

Perspiration causes acne. No, but perspiration is usually accompanied by an overproduction of sebum, the oily secretion of the sebaceous glands which can block or "clog" the pores. A blocked pore usually remains a simple blackhead unless bacteria get into the act, breaking down the sebum and the surrounding walls of skin cells. When this happens, the blocked pore turns into a highly visible infection.

Spicy foods make your skin break out. Very spicy food stimulates perspiration. In fact, people in hot countries, like India, usually eat "hot" foods, like curry, specifically for this purpose, since perspiration evaporates on the skin and creates a temporary cooling effect. However, spices also stimulate oil glands, and perspiration plus extra oil on the skin *can* spell acne.

See also CHOCOLATE, FRIED FOODS, NATURAL FOODS, TUNA FISH.

aging.

Senility and loss of memory are inevitable with age. Not necessarily. We are only now beginning to understand that many of the symptoms that we have grouped together under the general name of *senility* may be caused by a host of conditions other than advancing age. Truly senile individuals, victims of *senile dementia,* do lose mental acuity. They cannot remember things which have happened within the past twenty-four hours or so (although their memory of events long past may be unimpaired) and they are no longer actively interested in the life around them. The body and mind of the patient with true senility may deteriorate to the point where he is quite unable to care for himself, requiring the assistance of a nurse or nursing home environment for the most basic functions.

All the symptoms of senile dementia, however, may also be caused by disorders other than age. Tumors, for example, may cause the shaking hands associated with aging. Nutritional deficiencies, infections or drug reactions can cause loss of memory, vagueness and a disinterest in one's self and others. Once treated, of course, people whose senility-like condition stems from any of these problems, will recover, quite possibly to go on for years of active, healthy life.

Another thing which seems to stave off the loss of mental faculties is oxygen. It appears that both oxygen therapy and an exercise program designed to increase the flow of oxygented blood to the brain have, in some cases, been able to dispel mental fogginess. This may well turn out to be the reason why some people who exercise regularly or lead active lives seem less likely to end up doddery in old age.

Everyone gets fat with age. There is no doubt about the fact that middle age spread is a nasty reality, particularly for women who even though they were slim all though adolescence and young adulthood suddenly turn up chubby at forty. What's happening owes something to gravity, of course, but much more to hormonal changes. With age, the metabolism slows so that all of us, male as well as female, need less calories to maintain exactly the same weight. Fighting to adjust to a new calorie balance can be tough, and it's made even more so by the fact that even if the calories are kept in check, flabby muscles can make us look fat anyway. The only realistic solution (short of giving in) seems to be a sensible diet which (for women, at least) should supply just about 14 calories a day for each pound of desired body weight) and a sensible exercise program. And the key word in the exercise really is sensible since so many fashionable exercises like running, jogging and push-ups can put unbearable strain on older spines and joints, leaving the aging chubby person worse off than when he or she started.

With age, everyone grows "long in tooth." As we grow older, it is likely that all of us will lose some of the bone in our jaws to the ravages of periodontal disease. The loss of this bone causes the gum to draw up higher on the tooth, making the tooth look longer. And, even if we manage to avoid periodontal disease, the fact is that the gums, like other body tissues, tend to shrink with age, again making the teeth look longer.

Your muscles turn to fat as you get older. Muscles are muscles and fat is fat and they are two entirely different kinds of tissue; even the aging process can't turn one into the other. But, if you let yourself go, your previously tight muscles will slacken and you may gain weight. The result is what looks like fat in place of muscle, but it's really only fat on top of flabby muscle.

Everyone loses his/her teeth with age. If you expect to, the chances are good that you will. People who expect to lose their teeth anyway usually don't get good dental care and aren't conscientious about cleaning their teeth at home and watching their diet. As a result, there are some twenty-five million people in this country who have not a tooth of their own left in their heads. Another twenty-five million have lost at least half their teeth, and anyone who makes it past thirty without a single extraction is a rarity.

With the exception of wisdom teeth, which no longer fit properly in our smaller, more evolved jaws, all our teeth have the potential to last as long as we do. People usually lose teeth to decay or to periodontal disease which erodes the bone around otherwise sound teeth and loosens the tissues which support them. In almost all cases, The American Dental Association says that cooperation between dentist and patient might well have saved the teeth. If your dentist disputes that, you might consider another dentist. Perhaps the first one simply believes the myth.

See also, EXERCISE, GLAUCOMA, SEXUAL POTENCY.

air conditioning.

Air conditioning causes colds. Only viruses cause true colds, which are viral infections. But there are two ways in which air conditioning can cause allergic reactions which resemble colds.

In the first case, the swift change in temperature experienced in going from the warm weather outside to the cold of an air-conditioned room can cause the mucous membranes in the nasal passages to swell and "weep." This is called vasomotor rhinitis: the allergic person sneezes, coughs, and in general exhibits all the symptoms of a classic cold. Second, turning on an air conditioner which hasn't run in some time can blow dirt, dust, and, most important, mold spores through the room so that, once again, an allergic person shows all the signs of having a cold when what is actually being experienced is a run-of-the-mill allergic reaction. (Steam heat, of course, can cause precisely the same reactions for precisely the same reasons: a swift change of temperature and/or a fine spray of allergens.)

alcoholism.

Alcoholism is inherited. For centuries, it was widely believed that both good and bad patterns of behavior could be inherited, that the son of a thief would inherit a tendency to thievery, while the son of the noble would turn out, well, nobly. That, in fact, is the original meaning of the phrase "Blood will tell." See BLOOD.

Since alcoholism, or drunkenness, was regarded simply as a behavior pattern, it too was thought to be an inherited character trait. Twentieth-century research, however, has shown that the abuse of alcohol is a disease which can be traced either to conditioning within the family (in such families, the children are likely either to accept the idea that excessive drinking is normal or to reject alcohol entirely) or to a physical quirk, some inability of the body to tolerate seemingly "normal" doses of alcoholic beverages. Many "drunks," for example, get drunk on one, two, or three drinks.

In 1976, three researchers at the Bronx Veterans Administration Hospital and the Mount Sinai School of Medicine in New York discovered a specific abnormality in the blood which occurs only in alcoholics. This may turn out to be a diagnostic clue, showing well in advance which of us simply cannot tolerate alcoholic beverages. Since an abnormality like this may or may not be inherited, the possibility does exist that alcoholism, or at least the tendency toward it, may indeed turn out to be a trait inherited through the genes.

Further possible support for the idea that alcoholism may be an inherited disease comes from 1975 reports of two studies undertaken by Dr. Donald Goodwin, director of the Washington University Addiction Research Center in St. Louis. One study was carried out in Denmark and one here in the United States. In the Danish study, thirty-year-old adopted males were shown to be likely to mimic the alcoholic behavior of their natural parents, no matter how their adoptive parents behaved. (The study was conducted in Denmark specifically because Danish adoption records contain information about the natural parents' drinking habits. Of course, a psychiatrist might say that, if this information is available, it would allow the adoptive parents to precondition their adopted child. Knowing, for example, that the natural father had been an alcohol abuser, the parents might treat the child as a high risk, thus precipitating the behavior they fear.)

aloe.

The juice of the aloe plant heals cuts, nicks, scrapes, and burns. The aloe plant's juice is rich in oils which can have a soothing effect on damaged or injured skin, but there is no evidence to show that this liquid helps to speed the healing process. In his work at the Shriners Hospital Burn Institute in Galveston, Texas, Dr. Duane Larson has experimented with aloe, using the juice as a burn dressing. He found that it did keep the skin supple (which prevents burned skin from drying and tightening in painful scars), but that it wasn't any more effective than ordinary burn dressings. His conclusion: regular burn dressings are preferable.

antibiotics.

Take antibiotics with milk to avoid stomach upsets.
Antibiotics are designed to kill bacteria and may not discriminate between good bacteria and the bad ones. That means that when you take an antibiotic for an infection, it will also inactivate or kill the intestinal bacteria which help you digest and then excrete food. (How severe this reaction is depends upon the individual antibiotic. Some have a wider spectrum than others, which means that they affect more kinds of bacteria.) The result of this bacterial disruption can be simple upset stomach, diarrhea, or constipation, and in this case taking milk won't really make much difference. It won't add bacteria to replace the ones which have been lost, and, if your problem is constipation, you should know that milk and milk products may themselves be constipating. More serious, however, is the fact that the calcium in milk may bind and inactivate certain antibiotics, specifically the tetracyclines, including Achromycin, Aureomycin, Declomycin, Rondomycin, Terramycin, Vibramycin, and, of course, plain, generic tetracycline. And antibiotics which are not affected by plain milk may interact with other milk products. Penicillins, for example, are inhibited by, of all things, blue cheese. The point: check with your doctor before combining your antibiotics with milk.

Never take an antibiotic with fruit juice. Acid drinks, like fruit juices and some carbonated beverages, destroy some antibiotics, notably erythromycin. (On the other hand, the tetracyclines [see above] are potentiated—that is, made stronger—in an acid setting.)

Never drink liquor while you are taking antibiotics.
The list of foods and medicines with which liquor interacts—usually to the drinker's cost—is growing every day. Certainly it is now known that alcohol interacts with antibiotics just as it does with most other medications. It makes some antibiotics, like the tetracyclines, stronger, and others, like penicillin, weaker, and sometimes alcohol in combination with antibiotics can produce side effects such as flushing, hyperventilation and vomiting.

Keep your antibiotics in the refrigerator. Unnecessary.

In fact, dampness may adversely affect the capsules or tablets which keep best in dry, normal conditions at room temperature. They should, though, be kept away from extreme heat (like next to the radiator) and out of direct sunlight, since both light and heat can cause the medication to deteriorate.

Just to be safe, it's best to take antibiotics when you have a cold. Antibiotics, which are active against bacterial infections, won't lay a finger on the virus which is causing your cold. Some doctors give them anyway, to prevent complications such as sore throat or infected sinuses, but many experts say that it is always better to hold off on antibiotics unless they are specifically required. There are two good reasons for this kind of caution. First, most antibiotics have some adverse effects and sometimes these side effects can be serious. Chloramphenicol, for example, may cause aplastic anemia, an almost always fatal blood disorder. If the patient has typhus, which responds well to this drug, it may be worth risking the anemia to cure the typhus. However, chloramphenicol is totally useless against the virus which causes the common cold; nevertheless, for years it was routinely prescribed for this relatively minor complaint. The benefit to the patient was nil; the risk was enormous.

There is yet another reason to avoid unnecessary antibiotic therapy: bacteria become resistant to drugs. For a long time, many people thought that the idea of drug-resistant bacteria was simply a microbiologist's nightmare, but there are now strains of pneumonia organisms which do not bow to penicillin or which require massive doses of the drug, where once small doses sufficed. All in all, antibiotics are big guns which should only be used to knock off major diseases.

appendicitis.

Eating fruit seeds can cause appendicitis. While surgeons often find small bits of matter, including feces, in appendices which have been removed because they became inflamed, they rarely (if ever) find a fruit seed, like a watermelon seed or a cherry pit. Usually these small stones go right through the body.

A severe pain in the lower right side of the body means appendicitis. It can, but so can a pain in the upper right side of the abdomen, and sometimes the pain may be referred to a point as far away as the right shoulder. A much better indication of appendicitis is a blood count; if the white-cell count is elevated, it means that there is an infection present. Combine that with pain, nausea, vomiting, and a rigid abdomen, and you have the classic appendicitis picture.

apples.

An apple a day keeps the doctor away. According to the International Apple Institute in Washington, D.C., this familiar little rhyme (which has been popular in this country for more than a hundred years) almost certainly comes from an Olde English verse which runs: "Ate an apfel/avore gwain bed/makes the doctor/beg his bread."

Apple or apfel, this fruit really does seem to have a lot going for it although, if you want to be really precise about it, it won't keep the doctor at bay if you have a strep throat or even a bad cold. On the other hand, apples can help you digest your meals. They contain pectin, which increases the population of flora in your intestines. (Apples turn into applesauce when the stiffening pectin is melted by heat.) Some nutrition writers speculate that pectin can lower the cholesterol level in your blood. Apples also contain an abundance of the crude fiber hemicellulose, which helps to bulk up the waste material you excrete.

An apple is nature's toothbrush. For a while in the late 1960s, it really seemed as though there might be some scientific justification for the belief that munching on a nice tart apple after meals could cut down on tooth decay.

The theory went something like this: Apples taste acid and therefore they stimulate the production of saliva in your mouth. Saliva is alkaline, so it counters the acidity of the food you eat, cuts down on the nutrients such food provides for decay-causing bacteria, and, therefore, prevents decay.

Recent studies, though (including one reported in the *British Medical Journal*), have shown that the alkalinity of the saliva is more than neutralized by the acidity of the sugar in the apple itself.

As for the idea that chomping on a hard apple will actually clean your teeth, forget it. There's no question that chewing, really *chewing*, hard foods is stimulating for your gums, not to mention your jaw muscles. But even an apple leaves an acid sugar residue on your teeth and gums that must be cleaned off with (what else?) a toothbrush.

arthritis.

Arthritis can be controlled by diet alone. To date, diets rich in (or lacking) the following have been proposed as arthritis cures: Vitamins A, B, C, D, E, and K, fresh greens, honey and vinegar, celery, flour, starch, and sugar. But the fact is that food diets have no impact at all on the course of the disease. Neither do the vitamin-enriched or -deprived regimens, but it is important to note that Vitamins A and D can be toxic if taken in large amounts and should never be used without a doctor's advice.

Acid foods make arthritis worse. There is no evidence whatsoever that "acid foods," which usually translates out as citrus fruits, have any effect at all on arthritis.

See also BEE STINGS, COPPER.

aspirin.

Taken together, aspirin and Coca-Cola® can make you high. Among the raw ingredients used to create the flavor which we know as Coca-Cola® are the coca leaf and the kola nut. The coca leaf is one source of cocaine. Because cocaine was not a prohibited substance when Coca-Cola® was first invented, around the turn of the century, a lot of people have often speculated that the original formula, reputed to have packed quite a punch, contained cocaine.

Today, of course, we know that there is no coke in Coke®. Before they are used to flavor colas, coca leaves are purified and all traces of cocaine removed. Not that there aren't stimulants in cola drinks. There are. Two of them, ecgonine and cuscohygrine, come from the coca leaf. The third is caffeine, which is added to the drink in order to intensify flavor. Ecgonine and cuscohygrine may be new to you, but everyone knows what caffeine does. It makes some people jumpy and most people are simply more alert or bright-eyed after drinking coffee, tea or colas. (Two ten ounce glasses of cola contain about as much caffeine as one regular cup of coffee.) In addition, caffeine (in the form of a cup of coffee) and aspirin are the sina qua non of folk remedies for headaches. The combination usually works because caffeine helps to constrict swollen, throbbing blood vessels while aspirin soothes the pain. There is no logical reason why the caffeine from a cola shouldn't work as well as the caffeine from coffee. Or why it should make you any "higher," or more giddy.

"Take two aspirin and call me in the morning." Most people interpret this as the doctor's way of avoiding patients late at night, but actually it makes good medical sense. If what's bothering you is a fever, it will probably be higher at night. Aspirin lowers fever and so does a good night's rest. Pain too is often worse at night, possibly because when the distractions of the day are removed the pain demands more attention. Again, aspirin can be of real help, easing the pain enough to allow the patient a decent night's sleep. In the morning, the fever or pain may have disappeared. (None of this, of course, applies to true emergencies, such as appendicitis, and a good doctor usually knows the difference.)

Aspirin should be chewed before you swallow it. When you swallow a whole aspirin, it may lie against the stomach wall as it dissolves and cause (in most cases, minor) gastric bleeding. When the tablets are crushed into smaller particles, they dissolve more quickly and often don't have time to erode the gastric walls enough to cause even minimal bleeding. It would be better, however, to crush the tablets in a spoon than to chew them since in chewing you risk catching particles on your gums or in the lining of the mouth, where they might be irritating.

Aspirin cures a cold. Study after study has shown with depressing regularity that, while aspirin may relieve the aching muscle pains and headaches which go with colds and flu, it does nothing at all to alter the course of the disease. Ironically, however, scientists now speculate that, if you have a cold and take aspirin for it, the aspirin may increase your chances of passing your cold on to your relatives and friends.

Researchers at the University of Chicago reported in 1975 that aspirin appears to increase the amount of cold viruses that are shed in nasal secretions. This means that anyone taking aspirin for cold symptoms will be spraying more than the usual amount of viruses around the room every time he sneezes, coughs, or even breathes. Considering the fact that most adults catch their colds from the viruses blown by people who don't cover their mouths or noses when they cough or sneeze (people who do use their hands to cover sneezes pass the viruses along on their hands), healthy people sharing living or working quarters with a cold victim may wish to consider the advisability of putting a lock on the aspirin bottle in self-defense.

Gargling with aspirin relieves a sore throat. Only if you swallow the gargle. Aspirin is not a topical anesthetic—that is, it will not work if you apply it to the skin or mucous membrances. You have to get it into your bloodstream in order to get any pain relief.

To cure a toothache, let an aspirin dissolve against your gum. You'd have the same problem here as you'd have in trying to cure a sore throat with an aspirin gargle: aspirin just won't work as a topical anesthetic. In addition, there's the real possibility that you may burn your gum or tongue if you hold the acid aspirin in place in your mouth.

To relieve a toothache, you've simply got to bite the bullet and swallow the aspirin. But think twice about swallowing it if you are going to have the tooth extracted during the next twelve hours or so. Aspirin reduces the blood's ability to clot and people who take it just before or after a surgical procedure usually have more swelling and bleeding than those who don't. That includes people whose operation was a tooth extraction, as shown in one study of 32 dental patients reported in the *European Journal of Clinical Pharmacology*. The patients, each of whom had two wisdom teeth removed, were given aspirin to relieve the pain after one extraction and acetaminophen after the other. Both medications were effective against the pain, but the aspirin seemed to increase swelling and bleeding by about half.

Aspirin is one of the few drugs pregnant women can take without worrying about harm to the fetus. On the contrary, recent research seems to show that the use of aspirin during pregnancy may result in anemia, hemorrhages, prolonged pregnancies, complicated deliveries, and even an increased rate of stillborn infants. Researchers at the Royal Alexandra Hospital for Children in Sydney, Australia, compared 144 pregnant women who were regular aspirin takers (two to twelve tablets a day) with a group of control women who took no aspirin at all during their pregnancies. The aspirin takers exhibited increased rates of all the symptoms listed above; the control group did not.

All brands of aspirin are the same. Regardless of brand, all regular-strength aspirin tablets contain exactly the same amount of aspirin—five grains. But the aspirin, or acetyl salicylic acid, is packaged with a filler to make the familiar round tablet, and this filler may affect the performance of the aspirin. If the tablet dissolves quickly, for example, you'll get pain relief quickly. No aspirin will deteriorate in the bottle if the package is sealed, but a carelessly made container may open without your noticing it, so that the aspirin could be past its prime when you buy it and, badly-made aspirin may crumble in the bottle, so that you get a less than five-grain dose from an imperfect tablet. All in all, the same standards of quality control which apply to other products apply to aspirin. Even though the dosage is the same, the effectiveness of the pills may vary from brand to brand, and sometimes from batch to batch under the same brand name. Your best bet is a major brand name that sells out fairly quickly so that it is generally fresh in stock.

Crumbled aspirin is stale. If you find crumbled or broken aspirin in the bottle when you open it, that means that the tablets have been processed or packed carelessly. But broken tablets aren't necessarily stale or deteriorated. A much better test, in fact, the quickest and most valid one, is to smell the aspirin. If there is an odor of vinegar about them, they have deteriorated and should be discarded, as they will be ineffective.

If you take aspirin on a regular basis, eventually you will need larger and larger doses to relieve the same pain. There are a lot of pain killers—codeine, for example, or morphine—which begin to lose their effectiveness when taken over long periods of time. Your body becomes accustomed to them so that you have to step up the dosages in order to get the same relief. Aspirin, however, is not one of these drugs. No matter how long or how often you take it, it never loses its ability to relieve pain at the same relatively low doses. That is a major reason for aspirin's popularity as a palliative for people with chronic but controllable pain.

Aspirin substitutes are just as good as aspirin. It depends on what you want them to be good for. Acetaminophen, the drug used in brand-name aspirin substitutes, does relieve fever and pain as well as aspirin does. However, acetaminophen doesn't have aspirin's ability to relieve an inflammation, so it would not be as effective as aspirin against an inflammatory condition like arthritis.

Overdoses of aspirin substitutes aren't fatal. They can be. An overdose of acetaminophen can cause massive liver damage, and the symptoms of the injury may not show up for as long as twenty-four hours after the overdose, by which time it is almost always too late to repair the damage or save the life of the person who took the drug. Aspirin overdoses, on the other hand, produce symptoms—drowsiness, headache, nausea, vomiting, irregular breathing—which show up much faster, so that there may still be time to remove the aspirin from the stomach or bloodstream and save the patient.

athlete's foot.

Athlete's foot comes from swimming pools. It can, but it doesn't have to come to you. The disease we call athlete's foot (which doesn't appear any more or less frequently on athletes' feet than it does on others') is actually a fungus which thrives in damp places like the creases between the toes. If the skin there is cracked, somebody else's fungus, which may be lying in wait on the floor of a gym or the area around a swimming pool, can invade. But, if your feet are dry and free from cracks, you will be almost impervious to the fungus, no matter how many swimming pools you visit.

Sneakers give you athlete's foot. Sneakers have rubber soles and often are made of nonporous materials, which means that the perspiration from your feet does not evaporate. If your feet stay wet inside your shoes, the skin can eventually crack, and while that alone will not give you athlete's foot, it will make you more susceptible to the fungus which causes athlete's foot, should you come in contact with it. You can guard against this by wearing cotton rather than nylon socks and by purchasing sneakers with canvas uppers or with ventilation openings to allow air into the shoes.

B

※

baking soda.

    Baking soda is a "natural" antacid. Yes. Baking soda, whose chemical name is sodium bicarbonate, does relieve "heartburn" or upset stomach. And it is safer than commercial antacids, which may contain aluminum. According to Dr. Herta Spencer of the Veterans Administration Hospital in Hines, Illinois, taken daily, even low doses of some of these over-the-counter preparations can affect the body's ability to metabolize phosphorus and calcium. The result may be general body weakness, some pain, and a loss of appetite. Eventually, according to the report of Dr. Spencer's findings issued by the National Institutes of Health in 1977, the loss of calcium may lead to weakening of the bones (osteoporosis). Since there is no aluminum in plain baking soda, it does not produce this side effect. On the other hand, baking soda does have a few side effects of its own. Most notably, it can interfere with the body's ability to absorb a number of drugs, including tetracycline and some other antibiotics, anticoagulants (coumarin), aspirin, barbiturates, digitalis, and iron.

    Baking soda is a "natural" tooth cleaner. Right. To

use, mix the baking soda with water to make a thin paste. Actually, baking soda is best for removing tobacco or tea stains on a once-in-a-while basis, rather than for daily cleaning since it may scratch tooth surfaces.

Baking soda is a "natural" underarm deodorant. Works like a charm. It will not work as an antiperspirant, however, which means that it will stop odors but not the accumulation of wet perspiration. Interestingly enough, there are now commercial preparations on drugstore shelves which use baking soda as the "active" ingredient. They add propellants and sometimes perfumes though, neither of which does anything to increase the effectiveness of the baking soda.

A paste of baking soda and water soothes the itch or sting of insect bites. Yes. It's a nice, cool dressing, which is a lot cleaner than the traditional mud. Cornstarch works well too, and so does colloidal oatmeal.

See also MUD.

Adding baking soda to the water is a safe way to make green vegetables brighter. As other alkaline substances do, baking soda changes the chlorophyll in the green vegetables to chlorophyllin, a brighter green. However, in doing so, it can rob the vegetables of various water-soluble vitamins like thiamine and Vitamin C. Exactly how many vitamins you lose depends on how much baking soda you add and how long you cook the vegetables. So, while baking soda may make your vegetables *look* fresher and healthier, it may actually be making them less nutritious.

baldness.

"No boy ever gets bald, no woman and no castrated man." Aristotle said it first, and, to a large degree, modern science has proved him right. True pattern baldness (an irreversible loss of hair unrelated to any specific illness or injury) is an inherited characteristic. It is passed along in the male genes, and does not appear until

there is a sufficient level of testosterone in the body, which is why prepubescent males and castrated ones are generally immune. There are bald women, but their hair loss is usually temporary or, if permanent, related to physical trauma (burns which destroy hair follicles). In rare cases, a woman may suffer inherited baldness, always accompanied by an imbalance in sexual hormones.

Although the baldness trait is a dominant one, it may not show up if the level of male hormones remains low, so there has been some theorizing that doses of the female hormone estrogen could prevent true baldness in men. In fact, some hair preparations with estrogen have been developed. The results have been mixed: Estrogen, whether taken internally or spread on the skin, can have feminizing effects on the male body, and in some cases, genital cancers have been reported in men who used estrogen hair creams.

Tight hats cause baldness. Not true. True, pattern baldness is strictly a genetic gift. But a very tight hat can slow the circulation in the scalp and cause some hair to fall out. If this is the case, loss of hair will stop when the offending hat is discarded.

Tight ponytails cause baldness. Not baldness, but a reversible loss of hair. If the ponytail is tight enough it will simply pull the hair right out of the head. Loosen the ponytail, or discard rubber bands entirely, and the hair will almost certainly grow back.

Massaging the scalp prevents baldness. Massaging the scalp will increase the surface blood supply temporarily, but the blood supply (or lack of it) is virtually never the cause of baldness. Draw your own conclusions.

Baldness is catching. Some contagious diseases can cause a loss of hair. If you catch the disease, some loss of hair may follow. Temporary hair loss can also be caused by stress, which you cannot catch. Nor can you catch true, irreversible pattern baldness, which is strictly hereditary.

There is a special anti-baldness diet or vitamin. If temporary baldness or hair loss follows an illness, then certainly a nutritious diet can help to bring you back to par and, one would hope, can help your hair to grow back quickly. However, there's no known food, vitamin, or diet that prevents pattern baldness.

balsam.

The sap of the balsam tree eases a cough. According to the *Merck Index* (the standard encyclopedia of chemicals and drugs), the sap of the *Toluifera* balsam, which grows in South America, is the source for a purified, medically effective expectorant, used to loosen phlegm and ease a cough. North American Indians, lacking our modern techniques, used the sap of the balsam poplar straight from the tree, as an expectorant. The sap, though medically "dirty," obviously worked, for it is a part of medical folklore for any number of different cultures.

The sap of the balsam tree heals wounds. This is another hand-me-down from the Indians. Today, we use the sap of the *Toluifera pereirae,* which grows along the Pacific coast of Central America, in both human and veterinary medicine as a dressing to heal skin ulcers and other wounds which appear to resist ordinary healing.

baths, hot.

A hot bath can bring on a miscarriage. No way. However, not all women who think they are pregnant really are. If the menstrual period is near, it is not inconceivable that the hot water might help to start the flow. If that were to happen, a woman who had thought she was pregnant (but actually wasn't) might think she had suffered a miscarriage.

A hot bath is relaxing at bedtime. Like very cold showers, very hot baths (with water temperature between 98 and 100° F.) can be taxing to the heart. A medium-warm to comfortably hot tub, though, can certainly help to untie knotted muscles. Some people find that relaxing; others find that it simply sets them up for another go at whatever was causing the tension in the first place and, if that's the case, there wouldn't be anything relaxing about the bath.

See also SHOWERS, COLD.

Bee stings.

Bees sting "sweet" people. This aphorism, which is often used to comfort a shrieking child, does have some truth to it. Bees, wasps, hornets, and ants *are* attracted to sweet-tasting or sweet-smelling people. Hairspray, perfume, shaving lotion, or even some suntan lotions may be catnip to these insects (which also like bright colors and, believe it or not, flowery prints). To avoid being stung, don't use those cosmetics outdoors, and keep all food tightly covered. Watch the children to see that they don't wander around covered with ice cream, jam, or other goodies, which apparently appeal just as much to a bee as they do to you.

Bee stings sting, but, other than that, they are a minor annoyance. Yes, unless you happen to be allergic to the venom, in which case the sting can trigger a major reaction, even life-threatening anaphylatic shock. If you know you are allergic, keep a sting kit (which you can get from your doctor) with you at all times. Desensitizing shots may or may not be effective. Sometimes they too can trip off an allergic reaction.

If you are stung and suffer anything other than a minor local reaction, see a doctor as soon as possible. Hives, wheezing, tight throat, stomach cramps, nausea, or diarrhea following an insect bite are all signs that you need professional care.

Bee stings cure arthritis. No doubt anyone coping with the immediate pain of the venom which the bee injects when it stings is likely to forget, for a while, the deeper pain of arthritis or anything else. In addition, arthritis, like many chronic conditions, sometimes goes into a period of natural remission. The pain and swelling dissappear as if by magic. Should this natural remission follow a series of bee stings, the arthritis sufferer might well conclude that there is a connection between the two. However, according to the Arthritis Foundation there is absolutely no such link. Despite the fact that bee venom is being used as an arthritis palliative in many foreign countries, there is no scientific proof that it has any effect at all on arthritis.

See also MUD, TEA.

birth defects

Older mothers are more likely to have mongoloid children. The chances of a mother's giving birth to a mongoloid child rise from about one in 1,000 when the mother is 30 years old or under to about one in 250 when she is 35, one in 100 when she is 40 and one in 50 when she is 45 or older.

The reasons for this are still a medical mystery, but there are some plausible theories. The most popular one is simply that a woman's eggs, which are formed while she is still in her own mother's womb, are simply too "ripe" by the time she reaches her late thirties or forties, that they have degenerated so as to be more likely to produce a defective child. (In contrast, men produce sperm continuously throughout life, and thus far no correlation has been found between a man's age and the quality of his sperm although the quantity may decrease with age.)

Another theory is that the changing hormonal balance in a pre-menopausal woman's body somehow affects the viability of her eggs. A third possibility is the intriguing theory that it is not the woman's bodily condition which increases the chances of her producing a mongoloid child, but her sexual habits. According to Dr. James German of Cornell University, an older woman may have intercourse too infrequently to assure that the egg and sperm are fresh when they meet. Both sperm and egg retain their ability to fertilize and be fertilized for a day or more, but in that time their chromosomal material may begin to deteriorate. If that happens, the child who results may be defective in one or more ways.

How often is often enough to assure a fresh supply of sperm for a fresh egg? According to Dr. Robert T. Francoeur of Fairleigh Dickinson University, a couple who have intercourse every two days during a woman's fertile period in the middle of her menstrual cycle will be increasing the chance of optimum sperm meeting optimum egg.

See also GERMAN MEASLES, PRENATAL INFLUENCE.

bites, human.

A human bite isn't as dangerous as a dog bite. Wrong. Actually, it may be even more dangerous because few people take human bites seriously. The human mouth, like a dog's mouth, is a filthy place, brimming with all manner of micro-organisms, all of which can invade your bloodstream if someone bites you and breaks the skin.

Who gets bitten most often? You might think it would be dentists, but, according to Dr. Ronald Mann of the University of Miami School of Medicine, the likeliest victim is the policeman. Because human bites are often ignored, they result in a high rate of infection. Untreated, these infections may become so severe as to require amputation of the finger, the most commonly bitten part of the anatomy when the biter is human. (Dogs aim lower, for the legs, or a falling hand.)

black eye.

Raw steak is the best treatment for a black eye. The discoloration that we call a bruise or a black eye is caused by the bleeding that occurs when small blood vessels, just under the skin's surface, are damaged and broken. Sometimes, you can prevent this bleeding by pressing a cold dressing quickly against an injury; the cold constricts the blood vessels and stops the blood from spilling.

Raw steak is okay as a cold dressing, but a plain ice bag—five minutes on and five minutes off—is better and certainly a lot less expensive. Neither will have any effect on the injury once the bruise is out in full color, since by then the blood has spilled out under the skin. The cold steak or ice may make you feel better, but the only thing that will heal the bruise is time, which allows the body to clear away the spilled blood cells.

blister.

Never break a blister. If you are over thirty-five, you have almost certainly heard of the President's son who died after having broken a blister on his heel. Sometimes the President in the story is Coolidge and sometimes he is Herbert Hoover, but the results are always sadly the same. Actually, no matter who the President was, if his or anybody else's son died of a broken blister, what he really succumbed to was a raging infection which could not be controlled in pre-antibiotic days. Today we know that puncturing a blister, so long as you or your doctor uses a sterile instrument, can allow the thing to dry and heal more quickly.

Cover a blister with adhesive tape. A bad idea, since when you remove the tape you may tear off the entire surface of the blister. A much better idea, if you don't puncture the blister, is simply to cover it with an ordinary Band-aid and let nature take its course— which will usually be to create a small opening through which the liquid can escape so that the blister will dry and heal.

blood.

Blood is thicker than water. Actually, human blood is just about the same density as seawater, although it is thicker than fresh water. (See DROWNING.) The real meaning of this saying, however, is generally assumed to be that family ties are stronger than those in any other relationships. But it is interesting to note, for example, that most murders occur among family members, both blood relatives and in-laws. And anyone who assumes that "family feeling" is a genetic trait should take a look at research done by Harvey J.

Ginsberg, Sandra Hense, and Brian Bielfeld of the Southwest Texas State University.

The three researchers interviewed seventy children between the ages of three and ten. Each child was presented with a precarious situation in which he was asked to choose between saving a friend and saving a family member from some danger. Up to the age of six, the overwhelming majority of the children opted for saving the friend, who, as some of the children put it, was too small to save himself. After the age of six, though, the children usually opted for the family member, a result suggesting that the older you get, the more you become socialized to believe that society is right when it says that blood is thicker than water.

Aristocrats have blue blood. This obviously false idea is often thought to have originated in caste-conscious Spain, specificially in Castile. There, the nobles assiduously avoided the hot Spanish sun. Their skins remained pale, and their veins showed clearly through their skin. The veins looked blue, so the blood in them was assumed to be blue also. Out in the fields, the peasants were either sunburned or they had the naturally dark skin of the Moors. In either event, you couldn't see their veins clearly through the skin, and the blood didn't look blue.

Blood will tell. Originally, this meant that breeding, or "family," or hereditary manners would come through in a crisis when, no matter how many airs he put on, a peasant would behave like a peasant while a noble would naturally be heroic. Sometimes that works, and sometimes it doesn't, depending upon the character of the individual peasant or noble and having absolutely nothing to do with blood per se. But blood *will* tell—indeed it will sing like a legendary canary—if you know how to ask the right questions. A man's blood type, for example, can show definitely that he is not the father of a particular infant (although it cannot tell definitely that he *is*). Any number of diseases will show up in a routine blood examination, and there are now tests available to show a person's sex, race, and drug habits, all from the examination of a single drop of dried blood.

Bloodstains never come out. Of course they do. In fact, the simplest way to remove bloodstains from washable clothes is to throw the clothes into the washing machine right away. Dried bloodstains can be removed by softening them with oil (for instance, castor oil) and sponging with lukewarm water. If the stain is stubborn, you can add a few drops of ammonia to the solution, or you can dampen the stain with peroxide and leave the garment out in the warm sun to dry.

The idea that bloodstains are permanent probably arises from the psychological fact that spilling blood is a highly emotional act, no matter how it happens. When murder or foul play is involved, the impact is obviously much greater, and the culprit himself is apt to feel, like Lady Macbeth, that all the soaps and perfumes in the world cannot remove the damning stain.

See also HEMOPHILIA, SPINACH, WINE.

blood pressure.

Blood pressure rises with age. It generally does, but the cause may turn out to be an increase in weight rather than an increase in age. Studies of Indians in the Chilean Andes have shown that, just as with people in other cultures, their blood pressure rises as they grow older. At age twenty, however, the weight of the Indians stabilizes for life, and so does their blood pressure. The implication is fascinating, for, while medical science has known for years that a sudden significant increase or decrease in weight can raise or lower blood pressure, the importance of small steady weight gains has never been considered. Theoretically, at least, it appears that if you stabilize your weight you may keep your blood pressure at the same rate at age fifty as it was at age twenty.

body cells.

All the cells in your body are replaced every seven years. It is true that your body is a virtual hive of activity, with cells dying and being replaced every day of the year. The idea that it would take seven years to complete the whole body process has less to do with reality than with the magic often attributed to the number seven. Actually the process can be much quicker: for example, the entire population of your skin cells dies and is replaced about once a month.

body painting.

Covering a person's entire body with gilt or paint can cause death by suffocation. Balderdash, but so attractively packaged by Ian Fleming in his James Bond novel *Goldfinger* that virtually everyone who has read the book or seen the movie believes it to be true. Logic, however, will tell you that a person breathes not through his skin but through his air passages. So long as nose, mouth, throat, and lungs are in good order, suffocation is impossible. That's not to say, of course, that covering someone's entire body with either gilt or ordinary paint is a great idea. Aside from the obvious problems with skin irritations, there is the fact that ordinary paint is likely to contain pigments or solvents which can pass through the skin to cause systemic poisoning. Lead, for example, or turpentine, can cause long-term problems if applied directly to the skin, which is one reason why professional painters wear canvas gloves.

bones.

"I can feel it in my bones." Some people are inordinately sensitive to changes in atmospheric pressure. If they are allergic, overweight, chronically ill, or have diseases such as arthritis, they often are aware of changes in weather before these become apparent to the rest of us. While some of these people react with skin sensitivity or with a kind of prickling or "weeping" of the mucous membranes, a significant number feel the coming weather change in their joints and bones—just as the old saying indicates.

"Little old women" are the most likely people to end up with broken hips. True. After menopause, women become

susceptible to a condition called osteoporosis, which means that their bones lose calcium and become porous and brittle. There is some inconclusive evidence that osteoporosis is related to estrogen deficiency and some equally inconclusive evidence that the addition of Vitamin D or calcium in the diet may help, but, as yet, no one has been able either to prevent or cure the condition.

brandy.

Brandy is good for the heart. Like other alcoholic beverages, brandy is both a sedative and a vasodilator. It can help you relax and can also expand veins and arteries slightly so that blood flows more easily through them. Since these are beneficial effects for people with heart problems, brandy or cognac (the latter is brandy made from grapes grown in a specific region in France) is often recommended in moderation.

Of course, a moderate amount of virtually any liquor, wine or liqueur, would work just as well, but brandy and cognac are, well, so much more civilized. (NOTE: There is a listing for "Brandy" in the *National Formulary,* which is a guide to all the medication permitted to be used in this country. To qualify for the *National Formulary,* however, brandy must be made from the fermented juice of sound grapes and contain between 48 and 54 percent ethanol [24 to 27 proof]; it must also have been aged for at least two years in wooden containers. Commercially produced brandy, on the other hand, will run 40 to 60 proof and may be made from the juices of a number of fruits other than grapes, including apples, pears, peaches, and apricots.)

A nip of brandy takes the chill off. Yes, but only temporarily, and any other alcoholic beverage would do as well. The liquor dilates the blood vessels just under the skin, bringing additional blood to the body's surface. This causes a flush, or rosy coloring on the skin, accompanied by an immediate sensation of warmth. However, as blood is brought to the surface, the body loses heat. In addition, as the blood which has been chilled on the body's surface circulates back into the internal organs, it lowers their temperature, too. If you take your brandy indoors, you can eventually bring an equilibrium to this seesawing of internal temperatures, but if you take your nip outside in the cold—say, at a football game—you will eventually end up chillier than when you began.

breast feeding.

Breast feeding prevents pregnancy. While this one sounds like the quintessential old wives' tale, a study released by researchers at the University of Michigan late in 1977 seems to indicate that it may have some validity. The researchers, who surveyed 5,000 new mothers in Taiwan, came up with evidence that breast feeding tends to delay the return of regular menstruation—and also to inhibit conception. Among the mothers in the group who had nursed their infants, about 45 percent were pregnant again within six months after menstruation resumed. Among non-nursing mothers, the rate of pregnancy within six months was 65 percent. That may not mean much to American women, who have so many more sophisticated contraceptive methods available to them, but it could have solid repercussions in Third World countries where pills, diaphragms, jellies, and foam are either unavailable or culturally unacceptable.

Breast feeding prevents breast cancer. There is some evidence to show that the age at which a woman has her first child is related to her chances of developing breast cancer: the earlier the first pregnancy, the greater the "protection" against cancer. Since women who have their children young have generally tended to come from less sophisticated environments, where—again, generally speaking—breast feeding was more or less the rule, it is easy to see how the act of breast feeding could seem to be the element that offers protection. However, there has never been a single scientifically designed study which demonstrated any protective value in breast feeding so far as breast cancer is concerned.

Breast feeding causes breast cancer. There is no evidence at all to show that there is any correlation between a woman's breast-feeding her infant and developing breast cancer. Nor is there any evidence that a woman might be able to "pass" cancer on to an infant whom she nurses, although a number of animal studies have shown that the virus that causes certain breast cancers in animals can be passed along in the female animal's milk.

A breast-fed baby gets "immunities" from its mother's milk. Human colostrum, the fluid that fills the breast before the milk "comes in," really is chock-full of antibodies which can give the newborn infant immediate protection against some infections. In fact, various studies of premature infants, whose digestive systems are not far enough developed to handle non-human milk, show that those fed by their mothers on breast milk usually have the lowest incidence of infection. They are also less likely than babies fed on cow's milk or soy milk formulae to die while still in the hospital.

bruises.

Press a half dollar against an injury to prevent bruise discoloration. This works on the same principle as putting a raw steak on a black eye. If you catch the injury quickly enough and your half dollar or steak is cool enough, it may constrict small broken blood vessels just below the skin's surface and prevent the bleeding which causes "black and blue" marks. Actually, this one makes more practical sense than the steak remedy, since you are more likely to have a coin with you at all times. Ice, however, is a more certain remedy—that, is if you can manage to get it to the right spot fast enough.

butter.

Butter soothes a burn. Once a burn begins to heal, doctors usually use liquid dressings or creams to keep the skin supple and prevent scarring. However, the liquids or creams are generally sterile dressings which keep the burn safe from infection from various micro-organisms. Butter, which has been sitting around in your refrigerator, can't do that, nor can it have much effect on scarring when used as a first-aid treatment. All it can be counted on to do is to add a layer of grease and debris, which may well have to be scraped off again by the doctor. (A good rule of thumb is that any burn larger than a postage stamp should be seen by a doctor.) A much better first-aid treatment is to use very cold or even icy water. Plunge the burned area into the water and keep it there for a while; in some cases of serious burns, immersions may continue for up to two hours or more. The cold water (never put ice directly on the burn) appears to soothe pain and prevent scarring.

C

❊

---

calories

  Calories don't count. They do, of course, but they may not always add up the same way.

  If you eat more food and calories than your body can burn up in its normal course of activities you will store the extra calories in the form of fat. It takes about 3,500 calories to produce one extra pound of fat, so if you eat just 200 calories a day more than you can use up, you will probably gain one pound in about 17 days. That much is fairly obvious. A more subtle point, however, is that, while specific amounts of food may contain specific amounts of calories, the calories in some foods may not be as readily absorbed by the body as the calories in others. Calorie counts are determined by laboratory tests which show how food is digested and how much of it can be turned into calories, units of heat and/or energy.

  But the body doesn't always behave as laboratories say it should, and it is at least conceivable that some of the calories in such high-fiber foods as nuts, vegetables, and grains may pass right through the digestive system without serving either as sources of energy or potential stored fat reserves. One of the benefits of high-fiber foods, after all, is that they do help speed the passage of waste materials through the body by bulking up the waste and serving as a sort of internal bulldozer, pushing things along. It is interesting to speculate, that calories from different foods *are* absorbed differently; this would mean that we could eat, perhaps, 200 calories of corn for every 100 calories of ice cream, without expecting to gain weight from that "extra" 100 calories.

cancer.

A blow on the breast causes cancer. There has never been any connection shown between an injury, no matter how bad a bruise it leaves, and the later development of a cancer on the same site.

A lump in the breast means cancer. On the contrary, a certain amount of lumpiness in the breast is normal and increases with age. In fact, fully 80 percent of the lumps found in the breast turn out to be benign. They may be the small nodules of fibroadenosis, the slightly larger fluid-filled lumps of cystic mastitis, or the solid, benign tumor of fibroadenoma. All of these may be quickly identified by a doctor, and none have the slightest effect on a woman's general health or her ability to bear children. On the other hand, because the remaining 20 percent of the lumps in the breast may turn out to be malignant, any lump which does not disappear within a week after the menstrual period deserves a doctor's immediate attention.

Anything causes cancer if you get too much of it. This argument, which seems to be the logical extension of the motto "Everything in moderation," is often used by people who are too lazy or too frightened to make a decision about products which contain potential carcinogens. It is also used by manufacturers whose products contain suspected carcinogens to prove that "just a little can't hurt."

Of course, the argument is false. As a fast look through the *Registry of Toxic Effects of Chemical Substances* (published yearly by the National Institute for Industrial Safety and Health) will show, there are literally thousands of chemical ingredients which won't cause cancer no matter how much of them you eat, drink, breathe, or rub on your skin. And test after test by various agencies has shown this to be true. Of 132 pesticide ingredients in one test, for example, only about 10 percent turned out be potential carcinogens. The others might do people in in other ways, but even swimming in a non-carcinogen up to his chin won't give you cancer.

As for the "just a little bit can't hurt" theory, the scientific bottom line is that no one has ever come up with a lower limit for carcinogenicity. To do its dirty work, a carcinogen has only to begin to change a single cell in the body, and even if a smidgen of just one carcinogen won't do the job, a combination of smidgens certainly might.

Since we are all exposed to dozens of potential carcinogens day after day, and since the list grows as our testing procedures become more sophisticated, it certainly makes sense to avoid ingredients which may be carcinogenic and aren't absolutely necessary for our health. All of which is why it should be helpful, not frightening, to learn that *some* chemicals are potentially carcinogenic, for, in this instance knowledge truly is the power to eliminate these ingredients from our lives. To deny their potential danger by saying that *everything* causes cancer if you get too much of it only denies us the chance to make an intelligent choice.

Cancer is contagious. Some specific animal cancers, such as feline leukemia, which is caused by a virus passed between cats, have been shown to be contagious among animals. And there have been some suspicious groupings of human cancers, notably Hodgkin's Disease. But there is as yet no hard evidence to show that any human cancers are contagious.

Cancer runs in families. Certain specific kinds of cancer do seem to appear more often among groups of people closely related by blood. Women whose close relatives (mother, sister) have had breast cancer, for example, are often considered at high risk to develop the disease themselves.

It is important to note, however, that what appears to be inherited isn't the disease itself but the tendency toward it. That is, a woman whose mother had breast cancer won't inherit cancer cells from her mother, but she might inherit a particular type of cell or a specific chemical anomaly which would make her more likely to develop the cancer if she is exposed to a number of potentially triggering situations (a high fat diet, for example, is currently suspected of being such a trigger).

The same sort of thing may be at work in other kinds of cancer. Certainly genetic predisposition (or the lack of it) would go a long way toward explaining why one smoker develops lung cancer and another does not.

See also CATS, CIGARETTES, CIRCUMCISION, COFFEE, FLUORIDATION, FRIED FOODS, MENOPAUSE, VITAMIN A, VITAMIN C.

canker sores.

Canker sores are caused by too much acid in the body. Actually, a canker sore is a viral infection similar to herpes. It isn't contagious. As with herpes, you've either got the virus in your body or you haven't. If you do, it is likely to pop out during periods of stress. It has nothing at all to do with "acid in your system," whatever that may be. In fact, there is some evidence to show that increased "acid"—in the form of citrus juices and/or vitamin C—may actually help speed the healing process.

Baking soda, milk of magnesia, or other antacids can help relieve the pain of a canker sore. Yes, but not because they settle your stomach or lower that elusive "acid in your system." The mechanism is really much simpler and more logical. The primary infection of a canker sore is viral in character, but it is overgrown rather quickly by a bacterial infection, which is what produces that whitish sore. Bacteria and their secretions are acid, and the alkaline antacids can neutralize them. You can apply the antacid directly to the sore, or mix some baking soda, say, with warm water and swish it gently through your mouth.

Gentian violet cures canker sores. No, canker sores, like herpes infections, simply heal by themselves. Any dentist who smears gentian violet on your painful but harmless canker sores is simply humoring you by catering to your demand that he, for heaven's sake, *do* something.

canned foods.

It's dangerous to leave canned foods in the cans once they have been opened. Not at all. Acid foods, such as fruit juices, may pick up a slightly metallic taste from the can, but the Department of Agriculture says that has nothing to do with the quality of the food or with its safety.

carrots.

Carrots are good for your eyesight. Like squash, kale, corn, liver, and some milk products, carrots contain Vitamin A, which can help protect you against night blindness. Obviously, you need a reasonable supply of Vitamin A, and carrots, eaten once in a while, are a good source.

Too much of a good thing, however, will leave you not in the pink of health but, quite simply, *orange*. In *The Orange Man and Other Narratives of Medical Detection* (Little, Brown), medical writer Berton Roueché reports the strange results of two cases which turned up at the University of Tennessee College of Medicine in the early 1960s. The patients came in with bright orange skins. It turned out that they'd been eating too many carrots (which contain *carotene,* a yellow pigment) and tomatoes (which contain *lycopene,* a red pigment). The result was orange skin. How many carrots and tomatoes were too many? In one case, it was two cups of carrots plus two tomatoes a day. When the excessive carrots and tomatoes were eliminated from his diet, the patient's skin returned to its normal color with no lasting ill effects.

cats.

At night, a cat will crawl up to your face and suck the breath out of your body. Like other superstitions involving cats, this one derives from their legendary connection with witches and witchcraft. It may also have its foundation in the indisputable fact that cats do like warm places and will crawl up next to you in bed at night, perhaps even perching on your chest. They would be quickly dislodged by the movement of an adult body turning in bed, but it is not inconceivable that, should the cat crawl up on an infant's chest, its weight would be too heavy for the baby's body. The cat's body might, perhaps, be heavy enough to prevent the child from breathing and also from turning over to push the cat off. Should the child smother, though, it would have been from the weight of the animal, not because the breath was supernaturally drawn from its body.

Cats cause leukemia. Feline leukemia is a contagious disease among cats, and even animals which look healthy may harbor as many as 100,000 live cancer-causing organisms per milliliter of saliva. However, there is absolutely no evidence to date that feline leukemia can be passed on to human beings, or even that human leukemia is caused by a virus, as feline leukemia is.

caul.

A baby born with a caul has special powers, as does the caul itself. The caul is simply the inner membrane surrounding the baby in the womb. It is usually ruptured at birth, but a baby is occasionally born with the membrane intact, either around the head, or, less commonly, around the entire body. Obviously, neither the baby nor the surrounding caul has any special significance whatsoever, although the membrane was, for centuries, an important ingredient in many folk or black-magic cures and remedies.

champagne.

Champagne gives you a high faster than still wine does. You feel the effect of alcohol not when it hits your stomach but when it gets to the small intestine, from which it is absorbed into the bloodstream. The carbon-dioxide bubbles in champagne will send the alcohol speeding into your small intestine. So, all other things being equal—the number of drinks, the time that elapses between them, the proof of the alcoholic beverage, and how much you have eaten—champagne will indeed make you high faster than still wine will.

chewing.

Chew your food (35) (50) (100) times before swallowing. Though the magic number may vary, the idea behind this one is always the same: you'll get more nutrients out of your food if you "predigest" it by chewing it to smithereens. Of course, it's not true. The food you eat is digested in your stomach, where it is broken down by stomach acid and enzymes. The process does begin in the mouth (saliva is chock-full of enzymes), but you'd get exactly the same nutritional value from a chunk of meat swallowed whole as you would from one you chewed on for days. On the other hand, to avoid choking it always makes sense to take small bites or to chew your food long enough to break it up into small pieces. An inordinate number of Americans die at the table each year from choking on a piece of food, usually meat, which is too large to pass down the throat.

chewing gum.

Chewing gum clears your ears in an airplane. Sometimes it does the job. This is how: When a plane takes off, the pressure inside the cabin is lower than the pressure inside your ears.

As a result, the ear drum (the membrane that separates the external ear passage from the internal, or eustachian, canal) bends outward. To correct this, you have to let some air out of the eustachian canal. Since that opens into the back of your throat, the act of chewing gum and swallowing lets some air escape.

When the planes comes down, however, the situation is reversed. Now the pressure inside the plane's cabin is greater than the pressure inside your ears, so the ear drum is forced to bend inward. To correct that, you have to bring air in through your throat and up through the eustachian canal and then against the ear drum from the inside.

This is a lot trickier and less likely to work, but again chewing and swallowing can help. Blowing your nose, though, won't help at all and may even make things worse since the Valsalva maneuver—that is, pinching your nostrils shut, closing your mouth and blowing gently—can force mucus into the ear canals.

If you have a bad cold, it's obviously better not to fly, since you will almost certainly have pressure problems as the result of clogged passages. But that, of course, is a one-time thing. People with allergies almost always have problems flying, possibly because the constant swelling and "weeping" of the tissues has permanently narrowed the eustachian canals so that it is virtually impossible to correct pressure problems without some medical help. That usually means a regimen of decongestants and antihistamines specifically tailored for you by your doctor. It also means avoiding things which trigger your allergies a day or so before flying, and definitely avoiding alcohol, which causes tissues to swell, while you are in the air.

Chewing gum gives you cavities. It is certainly true that sugar increases the chances of your developing cavities because it increases the acidity of your mouth, encouraging bacterial growth and, sometimes, literally eating away your teeth.

But chewing gum, with or without sugar,* seems to have precisely the opposite effect. First of all, it increases the flow of saliva. Saliva is

*There is so little sugar in regular gum and it is out of the mouth so quickly—as opposed to hard candy, say, which stays in your mouth for minutes as you suck on it—that it really doesn't matter which kind you use.

alkaline and, since you haven't got any other food in your mouth while you're chewing gum, the alkaline saliva tips the balance in your mouth toward an alkaline environment, which is hostile to the bacteria and therefore kinder to your teeth. Second, the increased flow of saliva can actually strengthen your teeth. Teeth come into the mouth softer than they eventually end up. What helps to harden them is the constant bath of minerals (mostly calcium phosphates) which saliva gives them. Increasing the saliva flow increases the minerals. It's good for you.

Skeptics will be interested to know that all this is more than speculation. In one study, conducted in England, candymakers and bakers were told to chew gum steadily during working hours, while they were sampling their products. The result: the workers' rate of new cavities was cut almost precisely in half, a testament to the efficiency of a generally maligned confection.

If you swallow chewing gum, your insides will stick together. No. Like small seeds and pits, the chewing gum will simply be expelled whole from your body. (Its stickiness will be neutralized by digestive juices as it passes through the digestive tract.)

chicken soup.

Chicken soup cures a cold. Several years ago, some unfeeling cur of a scientist announced that not only didn't chicken soup cure a cold, it wasn't even very nutritious, since the chicken doesn't give up all that much to the soup.

On March 3, 1976, however, when the Food and Drug Administration's committee on over-the-counter cold remedies submitted its report (the committee had been evaluating cold remedies since 1972), Dr. Francis C. Lowell of Harvard Medical School, the committee chairman, said that chicken soup was "as good as any of them" in relieving the symptoms of a cold.

No one's saying—yet—that chicken soup "cures" a cold, of course. But, in 1978, tests conducted at Mt. Sinai Hospital in Miami showed that it does help to expel mucus from the nasal passages. At first, Dr.

Marvin B. Sacker, who headed the Miami study, thought that the soup's warm vapors might be doing the job, but it seems that the chicken soup worked significantly better than plain hot water. So the search for the real panacea in chicken soup continues.

chocolate.

Chocolate causes acne. Despite the fact that it has always been standard operating procedure for dermatologists to forbid chocolate to acne patients, there is absolutely no proof that chocolate ever caused a single spot to blossom on anyone's face (always assuming, of course, that the person who ate the chocolate wasn't allergic to it). In fact, the evidence more or less shows that chocolate has absolutely no effect at all on acne. In one study, conducted in 1969 by three dermatologists, 65 persons with acne were fed "chocolate" bars daily for about a month. When fed a real chocolate bar, 46 of the acne patients stayed the same, 10 got better, and 9 got worse. When fed a chocolate-flavored bar which looked exactly like the real chocolate bar, 53 patients stayed the same, 5 got better, and 7 got worse.

Chocolate is fattening. It really depends on how much you eat. One ounce of plain bittersweet chocolate (about one-third of an ordinary chocolate bar) has approximately 135 calories; an ounce of milk chocolate has about 147 calories. Plain, unsweetened, lowfat cocoa powder, like Hershey's, has about 54 calories to the ounce, and you'd use about one-third to one-half of that to make one cup of hot cocoa. So, reasonable amounts of chocolate could probably fit into almost anyone's diet. Some people even say it can help you to lose weight. The theory is that eating a single piece of chocolate before meals would help cut down on the food you eat at the table, but that's a risky strategy since one of the problems with chocolate is being able to stop after you've had that first bite.

Chocolate is high in cholesterol. Plain dark bittersweet chocolate has no cholesterol at all. The fat which makes it taste so rich is cocoa butter, which is higher in saturated fats than most vegetable oils but has no cholesterol. Milk chocolate, of course, contains cholesterol because it is made with milk, and even chocolate candies covered with plain dark chocolate may contain cholesterol if the centers are made with milk, butter, or cream.

Chocolate is "empty calories." Far from it. In fact, cocoa powder is a good source of copper, while plain bittersweet chocolate is a regular storehouse of such minerals as calcium, phosphorus, and iron, all of which are present in even larger quantities in milk chocolate. (One pound of milk chocolate contains 125 percent of the adult daily requirement of calcium and phosphorus, and about 20 percent of your daily Vitamin A requirement.)

Chocolate is energy food. There is sugar in chocolate candy, plus a pair of stimulants, caffeine (which is also found in coffee, tea, and colas) and theobromine (which is peculiar to the cocoa bean). Caffeine, of course, is a central-nervous-system stimulant; theobromine stimulates the muscles. Together, the sugar and the stimulants can give you an emotional as well as a physical lift, and, more important, the lift is often prolonged over a couple of hours because chocolate contains fat, which is digested more slowly than pure carbohydrates. That's why chocolate is a better source of energy than plain sugar candies or coffee, with or without sugar. During the Second World War, Hershey was able to create a six-hundred-calorie survival bar of chocolate which, while it couldn't sustain life adequately for weeks or months, was certainly good enough to keep a man going for a few days at a time.

Chocolate is addictive. Anyone who has ever tried to eat just one piece of chocolate knows how hard that can be. Some people say that's just because chocolate tastes so good, but it is also at least theoretically possible that caffeine and theobromine, the stimulants in chocolate, may be mildly addictive. However, it is only fair to say that there has never been any evidence that people who overindulge in chocolate experience the headaches or muscle tremors found among coffee addicts. And eliminating chocolate entirely from one's diet certainly doesn't produce the kind of withdrawal syndrome found among people who suddenly go cold turkey with coffee.

Adding chocolate to milk destroys the calcium in the milk. There is some oxalic acid in plain cocoa powder. This gives the cocoa a slight bite which is unpalatable to a lot of consumers. As a result, many cocoa powders are "Dutched," or treated with alkalis, specifically to eliminate the acid taste. For years, the belief persisted that the oxalic acid would bind the calcium in milk so that it could not be assimilated by the body. However, literally dozens of animal studies, some going as far back as the early 1940s, show that the oxalic acid in the cocoa has absolutely no effect on the calcium in the milk.

Chocolate ruins your teeth. Anything which contains sugar can have a potentially rotten effect on your teeth both because it is acid and because it provides nourishment for decay-causing bacteria. However, the less time it stays in your mouth, the less destructive the sugared food is, so, if it is any consolation, a chocolate candy which disappears fairly quickly, or a cup of cocoa, which goes down even faster, just may be less harmful to your teeth than a hard sugar candy which stays in your mouth for minutes at a time before dissolving.

choking.

People who are choking on a piece of food should quickly lift their arms over their heads while someone smacks them on the back. Lifting one's arms over one's head has no effect at all on a piece of food stuck in the throat. Smacking someone on the back will cause them to pull away from you and, even if you dislodge the food in the throat, the forward movement of the body guarantees that the food will fall farther back into the throat instead of out of the mouth.

The only sure way to save someone who is choking on a piece of food is to use the Heimlich Maneuver, which forces the food up and out. This is how it works: Stand behind the person who is choking and reach around him with your left arm, placing your left fist right above his waist, in the space between his ribs. Then bring your right arm around his body and use your right hand to push your left fist up into the victim's midriff. The effect is to push the diaphragm upward, creating a current of air which will send the stuck piece of food up and out of the throat into the mouth. Usually, the force of the air current will be strong enough to make the food pop right out of the victim's mouth.

If you are alone and choking, you can perform a variety of the Heimlich maneuver on yourself. Lean against the back of a chair and push that into your midriff as though it were someone else's left fist pushing into your body. The result should be the same: the food will come up from your throat, into your mouth.

When a small child is choking, the food can be dislodged by grabbing the child by the heels and holding him upside down. The physical aspects of this do make sense: by holding the child upside down you give the food a chance to fall out. But this should be done with greatest care since, with very small children if you swing them roughly upside down by the heels there is always the danger of a possible dislocation of the hips. It's far better to be certain that a child doesn't swallow large chunks of food or nonfood objects which can get stuck in her throat. In case of accident, though, you can resort either to the upside-down routine or the Heimlich maneuver, taking care to avoid injury to the child.

A small piece of soft white bread can clear away something stuck in your throat. Only if the piece of food or object which is lodged in the throat is small enough so that it does not block the entire air passage. If someone is having difficulty breathing, under no circumstances should he be given anything—white bread or a drink of water—until the food is dislodged from the throat.

cholesterol.

A low-cholesterol diet prevents heart attacks. It may. Cholesterol is a waxy substance which can adhere to the inside walls of blood vessels. Sometimes deposits of cholesterol can be so thick that the vessel is blocked and blood cannot get through. When that happens, the result is the classic heart attack. In some cases, simply cutting down on the amount of cholesterol in the diet can cut down on the chances of excess cholesterol adhering to and blocking a blood vessel.

But it is by no means a sure thing, because different people's bodies handle cholesterol differently. Some individuals, if denied cholesterol in the diet, will simply manufacture more on their own. Cholesterol is vital to the normal functioning of the body. (It is used, for example, in the production of sex hormones.) On the other hand, some people seem to be able to handle a surfeit of cholesterol in the diet with no problems at all. Researchers now theorize that this may be due to a difference in amounts of certain substances called low-density lipoproteins (LDL) and high-density lipoproteins (HDL) in the body. LDLs carry cholesterol around from cell to cell within the body. HDLs, however, carry excess cholesterol to the liver, from which it is eliminated from the body. The more HDLs a person has, therefore, the more excess cholesterol will be eliminated. So, if you have a high percentage of HDLs in your blood serum, the amount of cholesterol you eat may turn out to be irrelevant to your chances of suffering a heart attack.

On the other hand, it is only prudent to point out that as the American diet has changed in the past decade, with foods low in cholesterol and saturated fats replacing those with higher cholesterol and fat levels, the incidence of heart attacks has fallen for the first time since scientists began keeping track of such things. The thing to keep in mind is that while lowering the amount of cholesterol you eat can indeed be beneficial (for one thing, it's an easy way to lose weight since high-cholesterol foods are almost always more fattening), it is by no means a magic shield against heart attacks.

cigars.

Cigars (or pipes) are safer than cigarettes. Only because the cancers produced by these two are easier to reach than those produced by cigarettes. Cigars and pipes tend to injure the lips, mouth, and perhaps the upper throat. Of course, if you inhale, all bets are off.

cigarettes.

Cigarettes stunt your growth. To date, there is absolutely no evidence that smoking cigarettes affects the growth of the people who smoke them. However, if you are a pregnant woman, the cigarettes you smoke can affect the size of the baby you will deliver. Children born to mothers who smoked during pregnancy are, according to the American Cancer Society, smaller and more liable to be born prematurely than those born to nonsmoking mothers. In addition, a 1973 study from the National Children's Bureau in Great Britain showed that babies born to mothers who smoked during pregnancy had a 30 percent higher incidence of death than those whose mothers avoided cigarettes during pregnancy.

It takes years and years for cigarettes to affect your lungs. This is often said by teenagers attempting to justify their smoking. The assumption, however, has been proven false by a team of pathologists at St. Luke's Hospital in Cleveland, who put together a report to show that the damaging effects of cigarettes can be seen on lung and bronchial tissues of smokers still in their teens and early twenties who have only been smoking for a year or two.

Cigarette smoking keeps you thin. It may. Aside from the fact that the busywork of smoking—handling the package, finding the matches, lighting up, picking the cigarette up and putting it down, stubbing it out—can keep you just too busy to eat, there is also the indisputable medical fact that the nicotine in the cigarettes is an appetite depressant.

People who stop smoking gain weight. Nicotine not only depresses your appetite, it also speeds up your metabolism so that you burn food relatively quickly. When you stop smoking, your metabolism slows. You can equalize things somewhat by increasing your activity and exercising more. In time, your metabolism will stabilize once more, but in the first few months after you stop smoking you may, indeed, gain weight even if you do not increase the amount of food you eat. (Of course, some people gain weight for a simpler reason: they substitute food for the missing cigarettes.)

Cigarette smoke only bothers the person who smokes the cigarette. All cigarettes (and cigars and pipes) produce two kinds of smoke—*mainstream* smoke, which is inhaled by the smoker, and *sidestream* smoke, which drifts up from the cigarette, cigar, or pipe as it rests in the ashtray or is waved about. Sidestream smoke can be inhaled by anyone in the smoker's vicinity, and may be fully as devastating to the "passive" smoker as the smoke from the cigarette is to the cigarette smoker. Some research has shown, for example, that the levels of nicotine in a nonsmoker's urine rise with exposure to the smoke from someone else's burning cigarette, cigar, or pipe. And some people with inhalation allergies find that cigarette smoke, sidestream or mainstream, is a trigger that can set off serious allergic attacks.

Cigarettes are less dangerous for women than for men. This belief rests upon the erroneous assumption that women are less likely than men to develop lung cancer. In truth, as more women have been smoking for greater lengths of time, the lung-cancer rate among women has risen so that today it ranks second or third among cancers in women. In addition, researchers at the University of California in San Francisco have now discovered that nicotine appears to collect in breast tissue. They discovered the nicotine by analyzing the liquid normally secreted from the breasts of non pregnant women (ordinarily, this liquid, secreted in tiny amounts, is reabsorbed by the breast). No nicotine at all was detected in the breasts of nonsmoking women. Among the smokers studied, the level of nicotine in the breast was even higher than that in the blood. Does this mean that there is a connection between smoking and breast cancer? To date, no such correlation has been evident, but the researchers theorize that, as more women continue to smoke for longer periods of time, a correlation may appear.

However, there now seems to be enough proof that women who smoke cigarettes while they are on The Pill face an increased risk of heart disease or stroke to make it logical for the FDA to require that the leaflet which accompanies birth-control pills carry a warning to that effect.

Cigarettes aren't dangerous if you don't inhale. Like cigars and pipes, even the cigarettes whose smoke you don't inhale can cause cancer of the mouth and lip because they overheat and irritate those tissues.

As long as you aren't coughing, the cigarettes aren't doing you any harm. Cellular damage in the lungs, throat, and mouth can occur long before you start to cough. And bladder cancer, which has been linked with cigarettes, never causes a cough at all.

Filtered cigarettes are safer than nonfiltered ones. Not necessarily. According to a study done by Dr. G. H. Miller, assistant director of institutional research at Edinboro State College in Pennsylvania, people who smoke filtered cigarettes get more carbon monoxide in their blood because the filter prevents the smoke from being diluted by oxygen. The result is that people who smoke the filtered cigarettes risk dying as much as two to four years earlier than people who smoke non-filtered cigarettes. They die, as other smokers do, of heart attacks caused by the effect of carbon monoxide on the vascular system (it constricts blood vessels), and, of course, of lung cancer.

circumcision.

Circumcision prevents cancer. Statistics do seem to indicate that circumcised males have a lower incidence of cancer of the penis and that their female partners are less likely to develop cancer of the cervix. The culprit in both cases appears to be the smegma, or secretion which collects under the foreskin of the uncircumcised penis. Many doctors stress the fact that this secretion can be removed by careful attention to personal hygiene and that circumcision is not required. (There is no connection at all between circumcision and the possibility of developing cancer of the prostate.)

Circumcision increases sexual pleasure. The opposite—that circumcision decreases sexual pleasure—is also widely believed, but the fact, so far as we can determine, seems to be that whether a man is circumcised or uncircumcised has no bearing on the degree to which he enjoys sexual intercourse.

clay.

Eating clay during pregnancy relieves nervous tension. Among many lower-income women in the southern part of the United States, eating clay is a routine part of pregnancy. White clay is preferred, although women will settle for red clay if the white is not available. (Sometimes bags of the clay are sold in regular supermarkets; more frequently, the women dig it from road and river beds by hand.) What the clay does may be quite simple: it can fill the body's need for iron. Many poor women do not get a sufficient amount of iron in their daily diets—in fact, most American women, who restrict their diets to less than 2,500 calories a day, are iron-deficient—and the clay provides what's missing. It does it poorly, though, for the clay itself forms a filter in the stomach which blocks the absorption of the mineral.

If a mother eats clay while pregnant, her baby will be born free of "marks." The clay has absolutely no effect whatsoever on whether or not the baby is born with any birthmarks.

cleanliness.

Cleanliness is next to godliness. Actually, if you have allergic or dry skin, you may find that cleanliness is next to itchiness. Daily showers or baths can be much too drying for some skins, especially in cold weather, when both the weather and indoor heating conspire to rob skin of more moisture than usual. Many soaps, too, can add to the problem since they contain alkali (which wipes off the top layer of dead cells) and fatty acids (which are irritating). As for adolescent acne, frequent scrubbings with hot soapy water can further damage already sensitive skin.

cobwebs.

Cobwebs stop the bleeding from an open wound. The assumption here is that the blood will adhere to the strands of the web and form a scab more quickly, which is what seems to happen when you stick a "blotter"-type dressing, like a piece of tissue, on a shaving cut.

Whether it is the tissue itself or the pressure with which you apply it that helps to stop bleeding, there is no doubt at all that substituting cobwebs for tissues simply adds problems. Like infection. Spiders spinning their webs in the open or even in house corners create nets full of microscopic dirt and debris, none of which belong on an open wound.

As for a mysterious "Ingredient X" in cobwebs which might affect clotting time, forget it. Laboratory tests during which blood was poured into two sets of test tubes (one with cobwebs and one without) showed no difference at all in clotting times.

coca-cola.

Coca-Cola is an effective contraceptive douche. Insofar as any douche is effective in preventing pregnancy (and that's not very), Coca-Cola or any other soft drink will probably do. The drinks are acid and can make the vagina an uncomfortable environment for the sperm cells. In addition, the sugar in regular soft drinks can cause the sperm to explode and die.

However, douching with soft drinks or other aerated or carbonated solutions can be dangerous. The surface of the uterus, unlike the surfaces of the mouth, throat, and stomach, is covered with open blood vessels. If the soda douche is forced into the vagina under pressure, it may shoot past the cervix into the uterus, where it is conceivable that air from the soda might enter one of the open blood vessels on the uterus' surface, thus causing a potentially fatal embolism.

coffee.

Coffee makes you nervous. Caffeine is a central-nervous-system stimulant, and a study at Vanderbilt University in Tennessee has shown that the caffeine from just two or three cups of coffee can increase blood pressure temporarily, make the heart beat faster, change the rate at which your body produces hormones, and make you breathe more quickly.

However, like any other drug, caffeine acts differently in different bodies. While it may take just one cup of coffee to set your nerves jangling, the person next to you may be able to tolerate as many as three or four cups before feeling uncomfortably jittery.

Finally, you should know that cutting out coffee and caffeine abruptly can produce some wicked withdrawal symptoms. People who have gone this route have experienced headaches, nausea, and shaky hands until their bodies readjusted to life without caffeine.

Coffee is bad for children. Obviously, a central-nervous-system stimulant like caffeine is going to have an effect on a child's body and behavior, usually more of an effect than it would have on an adult's. Coffee, therefore, would appear to be out for youngsters. But, the major source of caffeine in a young person's diet isn't coffee, it's soft drinks. Most colas contain caffeine. As a rule, two ten-ounce glasses of cola have about as much caffeine as one good cup of regular coffee.

Of course, like any other drug, caffeine has its good points. It has been used to advantage in dealing with hyperactive children. Research at the University of New Orleans has shown, in fact, that caffeine works better and is safer in calming these children than most of the drugs ordinarily used. (Why use a stimulant for a seemingly stimulated child? Because many doctors dealing with hyperactive youngsters now believe that the hyperactivity is a sign of depression, not elation.)

Coffee cures a headache. Caffeine is a vasoconstrictor, which is to say that it can reduce the swelling in throbbing blood vessels in your head or neck. In addition, the mild stimulation of the caffeine can help to lift your spirits, and the nice warmth of the steam from the cup can help to relax your facial muscles. All in all, together with an aspirin or two for the pain (which the caffeine won't touch), a cup of coffee can in fact help relieve a headache.

Coffee keeps you awake. If you are one of those people who react to coffee with jangling nerves, then, yes, it will probably keep you awake, sometimes for as long as four or five hours after you drink it. On the other hand, just as it doesn't seem to disturb some people, it doesn't keep others awake, either. In fact, some people find a hot cup of coffee relaxing before bedtime.

Coffee sobers you up. Caffeine is a stimulant, so it may alleviate the depression alcohol sometimes causes, but there is no way that coffee can help to eliminate alcohol from your system, and you will stay "drunk" until that happens. It takes a while, but the only thing that really sobers anyone up is time.

Black coffee is a good diet drink. It doesn't have any calories and, because it is a mild diuretic, black coffee can help slightly to eliminate excess water and weight. But caffeine stimulates the production of stomach acid, and, if you drink too much black coffee without having any food in your stomach to neutralize the acid, you may begin to experience pains severe enough to be mistaken for those caused by an ulcer. For that reason, many doctors say that you should never drink your coffee black without eating something along with it. Some doctors take that one step further any say you should never drink any coffee, even coffee with milk and sugar, without having something to eat at the same time.

Coffee causes bladder cancer. A supposition of the early 1970s which has never been borne out by any scientific study of the effects of caffeine. However, at one time, several instant coffees (decaffeinated, as it happens) were made with a solvent called trichloroethylene, a suspected, though unproven, carcinogen. The solvent no longer is used in any of the coffees.

coffee, decaffeinated.

Decaffeinated coffee won't upset your sleep. It depends on your individual susceptibility to caffeine. Decaffeinated coffee has about 97–98 percent of the caffeine removed, but the remaining 2–3 percent just may be enough to keep some people hopping.

Decaffeinated coffee won't upset your stomach. In addition to the individual range of reactions to the minuscule amounts of caffeine left in decaffeinated coffee, there is also the new and interesting discovery that there is something else in coffee (no one yet knows exactly what it is) that stimulates the secretion of stomach acid just the way caffeine does. As a result, many ulcer experts simply warn their patients away from all coffee, decaffeinated as well as regular.

Decaffeinated coffee is safer than regular coffee for people with hypertension or heart disease. Since caffeine is a vasoconstrictor and vasoconstrictors (including things like the common decongestants used for colds and allergies) are *verboten* for people with vascular problems, the less caffeine, the better. And, since individual reactions to caffeine differ, even decaffeinated coffee can be deleterious to some people with vascular disease. However, there has never been any scientifically structured study which showed a connection between the consumption of coffee and the *development* of either heart disease or hypertension.

colds.

A cold lasts a week if you treat it, and seven days if you don't. Alas, yes. Anything that lasts longer is probably either (a) an allergy, (b) the flu, or (c) a bacterial infection, like sinusitis, on top of the cold. This last is the only instance in which it makes sense to use antibiotics in connection with a cold, since the antibiotic won't lay a glove on the virus which causes your cold, but it will knock off the bacteria causing the extra infection.

A hot toddy relieves the symptoms of a cold. Yes and no. It may anesthetize you so that you really don't feel anything, but there are drawbacks. First, the alcohol in the hot toddy (which is usually rum) will cause blood vessels to dilate and mucous membranes to swell so that your nose will be more stuffy and drippy than ever. Second, if you are already taking aspirin for your cold, the alcohol may combine with the aspirin to cause stomach bleeding. Therefore you should never combine the two, whether or not you have a cold.

Getting chilled means you're more likely to catch a cold. No. The chill isn't the cause of a cold, but simply its very first noticeable symptom.

Sleeping in a cold room or taking cold baths all the time can build up your immunity to colds and flu. No. On the other hand, sleeping in cold rooms and taking cold baths won't give you a cold or the flu, either.

Mustard plasters cure colds in the chest. Mustard plasters are what is known in the trade as "counter-irritants," which means that they sting slightly and make your skin red. This can make your chest feel sort of warm and will probably take your mind off your cold for a while, but it won't really do anything one way or another to affect the eventual course of the cold.

Hot buttered milk soothes the symptoms of a cold. Actually, it may exacerbate them. Milk and milk products, such as cheese and ice cream, tend to stimulate the production of mucus in your nose and chest. If you seem to be afflicted with continuous stuffy nose and throat, even when you don't have a cold, try eliminating milk products from your diet for a few days. If you find that you feel much better without milk, you may be allergic to it.

Cover your mouth with your hand when you cough or sneeze to avoid spreading your cold. This certainly looks and sounds like the polite thing to do, but, unless you use a tissue (which should be discarded immediately), using your hand to muffle a sneeze or cough is a sure way to spread a cold quickly. The cold virus lives quite nicely on damp surfaces, such as a glass or a faucet, and if you touch either after sneezing on your hand, you will leave your viruses there for the next person. Or you may spread your cold simply by shaking hands, using the hand you used to cover the sneeze. On the other hand, viruses sneezed into the air (as opposed to directly into someone's face), are likely to fall to the ground and lie there, out of anyone else's way.

Children with colds need bedrest. A child who needs bedrest will lie there without being forced. If your sick child is well enough to protest staying in bed, keeping him there may be a waste of everyone's time, since a 1965 study at Chicago's Children's Memorial Hospital showed that sick children used up exactly as much energy in bed as they would have used out of bed. In effect, the kids were "running around" on the bed. (Note: The figures on activity were derived by having the sick children wear pedometer-like devices on wrists and ankles, to measure their activity in and out of bed.)

You can break a cold by sweating it out. No, but some of the things which people do to makes themselves perspire heavily can make you feel better temporarily. Think, for example, of the pure pleasure of wrapping yourself up in thick blankets and lying out in the sun—or sitting around a steam room, letting the steamy moisture loosen up the mucus in your nose and throat (at home, you can use a small, room-model vaporizer to get the same effect). But once you leave the sun or the steam room, you'll still have your cold.

See also ASPIRIN, BALSAM, CHICKEN SOUP, DRAFTS, ELDER TREE, FEVER, HATS, WET FEET.

cold sores.

Sunlight cures a cold sore. Cold sores or fever blisters (the terms are interchangeable) are herpes infections, caused by a virus which lives permanently on your skin, waiting for an opportunity to break out into a sore. That opportunity may come when you are run-down and tired, or the virus may be set in motion by exposure to weather extremes: heat, cold, changing weather, or sunlight. Going out into the sun once you've got the sore won't change its course one whit, but there is always the possibility that spending a lot of time in the sun can trigger additional cold sores.

Cold sores are contagious. Individual susceptibility to the herpes virus which causes cold sores is decided very early in life, perhaps within the first few minutes after birth. If you catch the virus then, you will have cold sores on occasion for the rest of your life. If somehow you avoid catching the virus early in infancy, you won't. You can't catch someone else's cold sore (although, if it becomes infected, the bacterial infection on top of the virus cold sore can be spread from person to person).

color.

Colors affect your emotions. Yes, they definitely do. They also affect your bodily functions, like your heart beat, your breathing, and your temperature perception.

Ever since the cavemen first learned that the dark blue of night meant rest, blue has been associated with calm and relaxation. In fact, medically supervised experiments have shown that simply looking at something blue can slow the heartbeat and respiration and lower blood pressure as well. The yellow of the sun, on the other hand, has always stood for light, happiness, and action, while red, the hottest color of all, can make people feel warmer, more active, and sometimes even agitated. (The old injunction that a woman should wear red if she wants to be noticed is absolutely right.)

If colors are too bright, they can actually be so stimulating that they cause headaches. Very "quiet" colors, on the other hand, can make people feel cold. In one British study of the effects of colors, a workroom was painted gray and green while the workers were away on vacation. When they returned, they refused to work in the newly painted room until the temperature (which hadn't been touched) was raised.

color blindness.

Color-blind people cannot see colors. For the most part, that really should read, "Color-blind people cannot see *some* colors." By far the most common form of color blindness is an inability to distinguish between red and green. Some color-blind people cannot distinguish between yellow and blue. But only a small percentage of color-blind people are unable to see any colors at all, perceiving the world only as black, white, and shades of gray.

Only men are color-blind. In most cases, that is true. Color blindness, like hemophilia, is a defect carried in the X (or female sex) chromosome. Men have an X and a Y chromosome; women have two Xs. Since color blindness is a recessive trait, a woman who receives only one defective X chromosome will not inherit the defect. In order to be born color-blind, a woman would have to be the daughter of a color-blind man and a color-blind woman, or of a color-blind man and a woman with one defective X chromosome (if she receives the mother's healthy chromosome, the daughter will not be color-blind, although she will be a carrier who can pass the defect on to her male children). On the other hand, a man who receives an X chromosome with a color-blind gene will have no other, dominant "normal" gene with which to counter it. He will be colorblind.

Whiskey can make you color-blind. Alcoholic beverages can induce a form of color blindness, but it is strictly temporary and will disappear as the alcohol is slowly eliminated, naturally, from the body.

contraception

Douching with an acid solution like lemon juice or vinegar, or with salt mixed with water prevents pregnancy. Douching after intercourse is one of the least successful contraceptive methods, since at that point the sperm are usually well into the uterus and on their way to fertilizing any available egg. However, it is true that strongly acid solutions, like strongly alkaline ones, do make the vagina inhospitable to the sperm. For centuries, long before the more sophisticated contraceptive methods were devised, women knew that inserting a sponge soaked in an acid solution into the vagina before intercourse seemed to cut down on unwanted pregnancies. Of course, none of these solutions is anywhere near as effective as modern chemical barrier contraceptives such as foam or creams or jellies, which, when applied diligently and correctly, can approach The Pill in their contraceptive effectiveness.

The position in which you have intercourse determines whether or not you become pregnant. Some sexual positions which involve deep penetration of the penis into the vagina are more likely than others to deliver a lot of sperm right up against the cervix or mouth of the uterus. And the more sperm that reach the uterus the more likely conception is, always providing that the woman is in her fertile period. However, even positions in which the penis is not deep in the vagina provide sufficient access for sperm. In short, there is no sexual position known to man or woman which is guaranteed to allow intercourse safe from the risk of pregnancy.

A woman can't become pregnant if she doesn't have an orgasm. Women who think that they will not become pregnant if they avoid orgasms are placing their faith in a misunderstanding of their own bodies. The myth is based square upon the belief that an orgasm either opens the uterus so that the sperm can enter or releases the egg by shaking it loose from the ovary, the Fallopian tubes, or the uterus. None of these is true. Whether a woman has an orgasm or not has nothing whatever to do with conception, although it probably does have something to do with the pleasure or lack of it in the act by which a child is conceived.

Sneezing at the moment of orgasm or penetration or immediately after intercourse, prevents pregnancy. The idea behind this one is that the bodily contractions accompanying a hearty sneeze will either cause the uterus to contract and close so that no sperm can enter or will expel the invading sperm from the vagina. Alas, no simple sneeze, not even the paroxysms of hay fever, will have any effect on the woman's ability to conceive if she is fertile and the man is potent.

See also BREAST FEEDING, COCA-COLA, MENSTRUATION.

copper.

Copper bracelets cure arthritis. For years, the copper-bracelet cure has been regarded as sheer quackery, but there is now just the faintest glimmer of indication that it may not be completely so. Within the past few years, a Cincinnati chemist has shown that adding copper to aspirin increases the aspirin's ability to alleviate arthritis pain.

Now, if swallowing copper can affect arthritis, would it be possible for copper absorbed through the skin to do the same thing? In 1977, two Australian researchers set out to find the answer. Chemist W. R. Walker and psychologist Daphne Keats advertised for volunteers to test the value of the copper bracelets. Those who signed up for the study at the University of Newcastle in Shortland were given copper bracelets to wear for one month; at the end of the month, they were given new bracelets, which looked exactly like the first ones, but weren't copper.

The results of the study, published in a Swiss journal, showed that three out of every four people who wore the bracelets felt better when they wore the copper ones. Less than one out of every four felt better with the imitation-copper bracelets.

When asked about the experiment, representatives of the Arthritis Foundation replied that the study was unconvincing because it relied on opinions (such as, "I feel better," or "I don't feel better") rather than hard clinical evidence, such as reduction of inflammation or swelling in a joint. So the jury is still out.

corn.

Eating too much corn causes pellagra. For nearly a century and a half, American doctors preached the doctrine that pellagra—which shows up in such symptoms as sore tongue, cracked lips, red, itchy skin, and mental disorders—was caused by eating too much corn. In reality, however, the disease (which was prevalent among poor Southerners, both black and white) was caused by a deficiency of niacin or nicotinic acid, which is sometimes called Vitamin B_3. This nutrient is found in liver, yeast, milk, wholegrains, chicken, or stewed mushrooms, foods which were notably absent from the sharecropper diet. Adding the vitamin to one's diet immediately cures the disease, no matter how much corn one eats.

cottonwood.

Chewing the bark of the cottonwood tree can bring on a miscarriage. It may, for this maxim, which is widely recognized in the Deep South, where the cottonwood tree flourishes, is grounded in the truth that the tree may be host to ergot, a parasitic fungus. Ergot, which also flourishes on rye, can bring on uterine contractions severe enough to expel the fetus. In fact, ergot derivatives, used to strengthen uterine contractions during protracted labor (or to induce labor), were once used by illegal abortionists to end unwanted pregnancies.

Chewing cottonwood bark cures migraines. Again, the active ingredient is ergot which won't cure migraine headaches, but may alleviate the pain. Ergot is a vasoconstrictor which can reduce the swelling in blood vessels, which causes much of the throbbing during a migraine. Its medical derivatives are used, often in combination with caffeine, for both migraines and other serious headaches.

cranberry juice.

Cranberry juice cures or prevents cystitis. It's not impossible. First, any food, like cranberry juice, which helps to make urine more acid also helps to lower the incidence of urinary infection since most bacteria that cause these infections do not flourish in an acid environment. (Paraplegics and other persons whose bladders have to be emptied mechanically often develop urinary infections because the urine remains too long in the bladder. To counter this, they are commonly kept on acid diets.)

In addition, some of the drugs used to treat urinary infections work best when the urine is acid. The tetracyclines are an example of one such drug family. (You do have to know your medicines, though. The sulfonamides, such as Gantrisin, are not effective under acid conditions. If you are taking one of these and your diet is very acid, the tablets may be dissolved and the drug absorbed in your stomach, which means that only small amounts will make it all the way to the urinary tract where they are needed.)

Finally, cranberry juice contains benzoic acid, a natural preservative often used in foods to keep down the growth of bacteria, molds and yeasts.

crossed eyes.

Children outgrow crossed eyes. Not without help, they don't. Sometimes, the crossing may be minor enough to respond to exercises; sometimes it may require surgical treatment. Only your doctor can tell for certain which is the best course, but there is no question at all about the worst, which is to ignore the condition in the expectation that it will simply disappear on its own.

Dangling a toy or coin too close to a baby's face can make him cross-eyed. The baby may turn his eyes in toward his nose in an effort to get a better fix on whatever you are dangling in front of him, but, unless there is something wrong with either the muscles or the nerves in his eyes, they aren't going to get "stuck" that way, any more than yours are.

See also PRENATAL INFLUENCES.

cures.

The cure is worse than the disease. Whoever coined this aphorism probably was referring to the unappetizing nature of most early medications, which sometimes included such goodies as powdered bone, dried dog excrement, and blood. Or he may have been referring to early medical practices such as bleeding with leeches or cauterizing with boiling pitch.

But time has done nothing to alter the truth of the statement. With every medical advance have come "cures" which are either ineffective, unnecessary or downright dangerous. An obvious example is the "cure" for cold sores which was making the rounds a few years ago. The cold sore was painted with a red dye and then exposed to light. After that, it did curl up and disappear, but as it turned out, the treatment also caused changes in affected genetic material in body cells under or around the cold sore. It was, in short, potentially carcinogenic. Since cold sores usually disappear on their own in a week to ten days, the possibility of changed or damaged genetic material seems rather a high price to pay for a few days less of annoyance.

That same point could be made about any number of other "cures," some of which don't even work. Among them: X-ray treatment for adolescent acne (potentially carcinogenic), antibiotics for the common cold (worthless, and sometimes dangerous), hysterectomies for non-specific "female complaints" (bad medicine, or, if you will, malpractice) or tonsillectomies for some throats (useless unless the sore throat comes from infected tonsils). Before you take any cure at face value, be certain not only that it will cure but that it is necessary.

D

*

daydreams.

Daydreams are a waste of time. Although the daydreaming child or adult may look the perfect picture of a time-wasting idler, the truth is that daydreaming, like dreaming at night, can be an invaluable aid in problem solving. Psychologists have long known that people who go to sleep with problems on their mind often wake up with solutions which they may or may not remember having come up with in a dream. Daydreaming can serve much the same purpose; what looks like purposeless mooning can actually be a way of allowing the mind to free itself to come up with imaginative alternatives.

diet.

You need more food in winter than in summer. The rationale behind this one seems to be that it takes more food to keep you warm in winter than in summer. The truth, however, is that most of us are bundled up warmly enough in winter (or spend our time in rooms which are just as warm as spring or summer weather), so that there is no difference at all in our food requirements. In fact, we may even need more food in summer if that's the time when we do a lot more exercise.

Anybody can eat well simply by picking a variety of foods. Maybe, and maybe not. The variety has to include choices from the four basic food groups (meat and meat substitutes, such as beans; milk; grain; fruits and vegetables) not simply an arbitrary assortment of, say, meats or vegetables.

Left to their own devices, children will end up choosing a healthy diet. Not necessarily. It is true that people deprived of one nutrient or another will attempt to obtain it somehow. Persons whose diet is deficient in iron, for example, will sometimes stuff clay or dirt into their mouths. But the deficiency has to be extreme to trigger this kind of response, and, luckily, most children have not reached that stage. Left to their own devices, they will head for foods which taste good, and, although preferences may vary with the individual, a child's ending up with a balanced diet would be more or less a matter of pure luck.

Athletes need a steak-and-potatoes diet. The old idea of the high-protein diet, with most of the protein coming from red meat, has fallen into disrepute in recent years. For one thing, the protein derived from red meat carries with it the unwelcome burden of high fat and cholesterol. For another, it is questionable whether athletes need a diet any different from that which promotes good health in the rest of us, which is to say a normal, well-balanced one. (In other words, athletes may need more calories, but the foods they eat should be the same.) And most interesting of all is our relatively new understanding of the importance of carbohydrates in the diet. It is carbohydrates which are metabolized into glycogen in muscles and liver, and it is glycogen which gives us all, athletes included, that "extra energy" for the long push. By all standards then, a diet rich in carbohydrates and non-animal proteins (such as beans-and-rice) is the best one.

Eating meat makes people warlike. There is no histori-cal evidence whatsoever to prove that vegetarians are, en masse, less aggressive than meat eaters, although some vegetarians may actually be more peaceable than some carnivores. However, four researchers at Albert Einstein School of Medicine and Rockefeller University, both in New York, have come up with some tentative evidence to show that depriving laboratory rats of tryptophan, an amino acid found in milk and meat, among other foods, does make them more aggressive. Rats on a tryptophan-deficient diet began to kill mice without regard to whether they (the rats) were hungry or not. Ordinarily, of course, animals do not kill unless they are hungry, and they stop as soon as they have fed.

An examination of the rats' brain chemistry showed that depriving them of tryptophan produced a decrease of about 40 percent in the serotonin in their brains. Serotonin is a chemical transmitter, which carries signals from the brain to the other parts of the body, and the researchers theorize that the cells which produce serotonin normally inhibit warlike behavior, at least among rats. Therefore, eating meat, which, as noted, contains tryptophan, might actually keep the rats more peaceful.

A high-protein diet is the most healthful one. Perhaps not. In studies with laboratory rats conducted at the Fox Chase Cancer Center in Philadelphia and at Rijks University in the Nether-lands, the animals were allowed to eat unlimited amounts of one of three diets, the only difference among the diets being the amount of protein they contained. The rats died of natural causes at ages ranging from 317 to 1,026 days, which is a relatively normal range of life spans for laboratory rats. The rats that lived the longest, however, were those that ate a high-protein diet early in life, ate reasonable amounts (did not overeat) during adolescence, and ate a low-protein diet in adulthood.

Never eat more than one protein food at a meal. Different proteins are digested at different rates, and if you eat more than one of these foods something will remain undigested in your stomach. The truth is that you should often eat more than one protein-containing food at the same time to get the best nutritional bargain. For example, some grains and beans contain incomplete protein complements; by combining them in one dish (such as beans-and-rice) you get your full dose of protein. Even complete protein foods, like milk and cheese, work better in combination with some incomplete protein foods, like bread or pasta (which is why macaroni and cheese is a good nutritional bet).

dieting.

Dieters should avoid carbohydrates and starchy foods. Not necessarily. There are about 9 calories in an ounce of fat, 4 or 5 in an ounce of protein or carbohydrates. It's possible, therefore, that carbohydrates and starchy foods like noodles, bread, and potatoes can have less calories, ounce for ounce, than that diet standard, the steak. The reason is simple: the steak has fat (not to mention cholesterol) in it; the bread and potatoes do not. You can even use foods like bread, grains, and beans to give you proteins without fat. The ordinary peasant fare of beans-and-rice is a complete protein dish with none of the fat and cholesterol found in red-meat protein, and there are any number of such combinations of vegetable proteins which can be substituted for meat on a reducing diet.

"It isn't eating that makes you fat; it's swallowing." The possibility now exists that you may someday be able to eat—and swallow—anything you wish without gaining a single ounce. Researchers at the University of Illinois have discovered that a substance called perfluoroctyl bromide (which coats the stomach and was originally being tested as a means of preventing death by absorption of an overdose of drugs) also has the power to block the absorption of calories from food. The substance, when fed to rats, kept up to 90 percent of the calories in the food they ate from being absorbed into the body. (Naturally it also kept the rats from getting the vitamins and minerals out of their food.) It has not yet been tested on human beings, but who knows? In ten or twenty years, there may be a

container of perfluoroctyl bromide on every dieter's table, right along with the salt shaker.

See also CALORIES.

doctors.

Doctors cannot operate on members of their own family. There is no regulation, legal or otherwise, which prevents doctors from operating on or treating members of their own families. Common sense, however, seems to indicate that in many situations emotional complications might keep some doctors from doing their best work when a member of the family is involved. On the other hand, some doctors might do even better than usual, so the decision is usually one that the doctor makes for himself.

Doctors are less afraid of death that most of us are. Not true. Although doctors are generally expected to remain coolly detached from the drama of the life and death struggles with which they deal, the fact of the matter is that they face death with the same mixture of fear, anger, courage and foolishness that the rest of us do. In one study of physicians' attitudes toward death, psychiatrist Herman Feifel found that doctors, while they thought less about death than did a control group of patients, were more afraid of it than the patients were.

drafts.

Drafts cause colds. Not unless they blow some cold viruses your way. Like air conditioning, drafts or other swift changes in temperature may trigger allergic reactions in some susceptible persons, but never the viral infection we call a cold.

See also AIR CONDITIONING.

Drafts cause muscular cramps or "charley horse." It is possible that a sudden chilling can cause a muscle to go into spasm—

that is, to cramp. The condition can be relieved quickly either by warming things up or by keeping the muscle moving.

dreams.

Nobody dreams in color. Sure we do; it's just that few people are trained to remember dreams in their entirety, and what little one does recall usually centers around the most important part of the dream, which is to say, the action not the color. You can train yourself to remember your dreams by writing them down the minute you wake up (or as soon as you can handle a pencil), and, if you do, you may be surprised to find that you can remember the colors in your dreams, as well as what happened.

Eating before you go to sleep causes nightmares. It depends upon what you eat. According to research done at St. George's Medical School in London, a normally balanced dinner, which included ordinary amounts of proteins, fats, and carbohydrates, produced a normal night's sleep. On the other hand, a meal high in carbohydrates and low in fat led to a night filled with active dreaming (so did a meal high in fat and low in carbohydrates). In other words, a heavy starchy or fatty meal (or snack just before bedtime) probably means a good night of dreams afterward; an ordinary light dinner probably means you'll sleep soundly.

Dreams foretell the future. Sometimes they appear to, but it oftens turns out that the dream which foretells the future is really a self-fulfilling prophecy. That is, the dreamer, working with known facts, sets up a situation and proceeds to follow it through to a logical or at least hoped-for conclusion in the dream. Once awake, the dreamer either consciously or unconsciously begins to follow the path taken in the dream, with the result that the outcome may, time after time, be the same as it was in the dream. Ergo, the dream "foretold the future."

drowning.

Drowning people come up for air twice before "going down for the third time." This is a neat formula, all right. It just isn't a true one. The human body will bob to the surface just as long as there is gas enough in the body to make it buoyant in the water. The gas in question can be the air in a living person's lungs, or it can be the gases formed by decomposition after death (which is why it is almost impossible to keep a corpse from rising out of the water where it may have been hidden—unless, of course, you put its feet in cement). The more water you swallow, the more air or gas you are apt to displace from the lungs, so if you manage to keep your head above water and water out of your mouth you can stay afloat almost indefinitely. People who bob up and down, however, are virtually certain to swallow water, perhaps even enough to keep them from coming up more than twice.

People drown more quickly in fresh water than in salt. It is impossible to point to any scientifically managed study which would show this to be true, but there is enough scientific truth in it to make it a theoretical possibility. The operant physical principle is osmosis. Osmosis occurs when liquids of different densities, on opposite sides of a permeable or passable membrane, flow toward each other through the membrane so as to equalize the densities of the liquids on either side.

If you swallow or inhale salt water, it would pass more slowly through the permeable membranes of your stomach, lungs, and blood vessels than fresh water because salt water is about equal in density to blood and body fluids. The fresh water is less dense than these fluids and so, theoretically at least, will flow faster through the membranes, diluting your blood and drowning you.

E

eating habits.

Breakfast is the most important meal of the day. Eating habits, like sleep patterns, are pretty much an individual affair, and attempts to make people conform to such neat formulas as this one about breakfast usually fail. So long as you get the proper amount of nutrients each day, it doesn't really matter *when* you get them. Ordinarily, we each respond to the dictates of an inner "clock" in choosing the times of day set aside for meals, for eating is usually a response to the body's signal that it needs food, and one of the clearest signals of a need for food is a drop in temperature. People whose temperature is lower in the morning will usually feel hungry then, while people who maintain a warmer temperature coming out of a night's sleep will feel hungry slightly later in the day. Interestingly enough, many people who start eating early in the morning slow down later in the day, when those who started later are just revving up, and the conflict in body schedules between a late and an early starter can be just as devastating at the dinner table as it is at bedtime.

Eating between meals is bad for you. The corollary of this, of course, is that the healthiest way to get your daily food is in three regular and balanced meals. It sounds logical, but the truth is that the evidence is mixed. With laboratory rats, short-term studies have shown that, when feeding is limited to one specific two-hour period each day, the rats' bodies work much more efficiently turning carbohydrates into fat and thus into energy. Rats which were fed at specific times also tended to eat about 20-25 percent less than their cohorts who were allowed to nibble all day long.

But human beings are less easily manipulated, and in many instances may do better (insofar as both diet and general health are concerned) on four, five or six small meals a day. People with ulcers and stomach disorders do well on a schedule like that with small meals, usually spaced three hours or so apart. But the surprise is that dieters may also do better on small meals taken frequently. The trick is to "balance" the day, not the meals, so that the same amount of food (or lack of it) is spread out over the waking hours and the dieter is not forced to become frantic about food.

Eating frequent small meals also keeps the body's energy level constant, but it may make trouble for your teeth. It's a chore to clean your teeth after every meal, but if you don't, eating frequently can have some effect on dental health, raising the rate of cavities or causing the formation of more plaque than usual. It's a compromise: frequent meals require frequent brushing; less frequent meals, less frequent brushing. Which one do you prefer?

eczema.

Eczema is catching. No matter how miserable it looks, eczema simply can't be passed on from one person to another since it is an individual body's reaction to a particular irritant or stimulus, which might not affect another body at all. Of course, if the eczema is infected, the infection can be passed around.

Eczema is a child's disease. Actually, eczema can pop up at any time in your life. In fact, men over forty are, for some as yet unknown reason, particularly prone to patches of eczema on the back of the legs or around the middle.

elder tree.

Tea made from the leaves and flowers of the elder tree cures a cold. The leaves and flowers of the elder tree, or *Sambucus,* contain tannin, which is a diuretic, as well as volatile oils, resins, and mucilage, which may also be diuretic as well as diaphoretic (perspiration inducing). The idea that the tea could cure a cold arose from its ability to eliminate water from the body; in most cultures, it is assumed that profuse sweating and/or urination can help you get rid of a cold. Not true, although you may enjoy the warm tea anyway.

epilepsy.

Epilepsy is hereditary. Epilepsy, or an epileptic seizure, is the result of a momentary imbalance in the electrical activity of the brain. This imbalance may be caused by brain damage resulting from injury, chemical imbalance, infectious diseases, fever, brain tumors, and, sometimes, poisons. Because brain injury may also occur before or during birth, some babies are born epileptics. But, so far as we know, their affliction is *congenital* (which means that it is acquired at birth or during gestation) but not *hereditary* (which refers to characteristics which are passed from one individual to another through the genes).

Epileptics are mentally retarded. Epileptics may be retarded, but so may people who have never had epilepsy. Epilepsy has no relationship at all to a person's intelligence, and epileptics may be intelligent, average, or stupid, just like the rest of us.

You can stop an epileptic seizure by dashing cold water in the victim's face. Once a seizure has begun, nothing you do can stop it from running its course. And, throwing cold water on an epileptic can be dangerous, because the water may be inhaled into the lungs and cause choking.

***During seizures, epileptics should be restrained—
forcibly, if necessary.*** Some seizures are so mild that no one other
than the epileptic will know they have occurred. The visible seizure,
however, can be disturbing to bystanders, who may assume that the
epileptic will hurt himself or become violent. Unfortunately, that is
more likely to occur if one attempts to restrain the seizure victim, who,
feeling the restraint, can struggle strongly enough to injure both
himself and the person doing the restraining. The safest course, for
both the epileptic and the bystander, is simply to make sure that the
seizure victim doesn't injure himself in falling and then allow the
seizure to run its normal course.

***During an epileptic seizure, you should put some-
thing between the victim's teeth so that she won't bite her
tongue.*** If you can insert a soft object, like a handkerchief, between the
teeth without forcing, fine. Never insert a hard object like a pencil,
however, and never attempt to force open an epileptic's jaw. You
might trigger muscle contractions serious enough to break her teeth.

exercise.

Exercise (or sports) makes a woman's muscles bulge.
Muscular development is a matter of genetic programming and body
type. A woman with a "feminine"-type frame will virtually never
develop the bulgy muscles associated with a male weight lifter's, no
matter how long or how hard she exercises. The explanation is
simple. Hormones limit the development of female muscles; both men
and woman have the testosterone which allows muscles to grow, but
women have more estrogen than men, and estrogen inhibits the
growth of thick, ropy muscles. Therefore, a "well-muscled" woman
will still be smoother and more compact than a "well-muscled" man.

***Women who "overtrain" their bodies have trouble
delivering babies.*** Women with well-exercised muscles actually
have an easier time of it in labor, always provided that they have a
sufficiently wide pelvic structure. Often athletes who have a difficult

time with delivery have problems because they have narrow pelvic girdles which work well on the athletic field but are less suited for labor. The problem, if one exists, is always body type. It has nothing whatsoever to do with athletic development.

However, women who train strenuously enough so that the percentage of fat in their bodies drops below 15 percent (the normal female's body weight is 18 to 25 percent fat) often experience interruptions in their menstrual cycles. They may skip a period now and again, or menstruation may stop entirely as long as they maintain their "training" weight. The problem is by no means restricted to athletes; it is common also among ballet dancers, whose art demands that they streamline their bodies to a degree counter to the biological norm, and among fashion models who do the same thing.

The effect appears to be temporary. When the women gain weight, and fat, menstruation returns on a regular schedule.

Never drink liquids while exercising. The idea behind this one seems to be that drinking while exercising or engaging in such strenuous activities as tennis, say, or football, bloats the body and makes the athlete less efficient. The truth, however, is that the body loses water very fast during strenuous activities and, if this water is not replaced, dehydration follows. The athlete can keel over suddenly in a dead faint—and in rare cases might even die—if the missing liquids are not replaced. So if you are thirsty on the playing field, drink up.

Never drink ice water while exercising. Ice water has the same effect on your stomach muscles that it does on all other muscles, which is to say that it can cause them to go into spasm. It can do this while you are at rest as well as while you are exercising, which is why people with spastic colons are usually advised to avoid iced drinks. (Hot drinks can also be irritating.) The best bet for an athlete is medium-cool water, as needed.

You can't lose weight by exercising. So long as you don't go from the exercise to the table, you really can burn off calories by walking (5.2 calories per minute), bicycle riding (8.2 calories per minute), running (19.4 calories per minute) and swimming (11.4 calories per minute). Serious athletes like boxers, dancers, and football players have been known to drop five pounds in a night (or day) of playing, but much of that drastic loss is water, which comes right back.

The best exercise is the kind that helps you "work up a good sweat." Exercise heats up your body, sometimes so much that, if you couldn't dissipate the extra heat, your internal temperature might rise by as much as ten full degrees. If that happened, you would run into all the side effects of a bad fever: nausea, dizziness, dehydration, and, possibly, collapse. Fortunately, the body has two ways in which to dissipate heat before things reach a desperate pass. First, the surface blood vessels, right under your skin, dilate so that more blood can be brought right up to the skin's surface and cooled before it circulates back through the body. Second, the sweat glands begin to produce moisture, which evaporates on the skin, lowering your temperature somewhat. If this production of sweat is excessive, you may find that you have lost some weight after your exercise session, which is probably why it is regarded as a desirable thing. However, the water weight lost during perspiration comes back fast and losing weight that way is not worth the stress such overheating puts on your body.

The best exercise leaves you slightly out of breath when you are done. Yes and no. It is rarely understood, for example, that walking, just plain walking, can be adequate exercise if it is done consistently and for long enough periods of time. Walking two or three miles a day will exercise virtually every muscle in your body, including your eye muscles (you swing your eyes from side to side as you walk down a street, don't you?) without getting you out of breath at all. On the other hand, a strenuous period of intense muscle exercise daily can leave you slightly out of breath when you are done. Your breathing and heartbeat should return to normal within ten minutes at the most, however. If that doesn't happen, you are doing the wrong exercises or exercising beyond your capacity, and that can backfire on you, tiring you out so as to nullify all the good effects of the exercise session.

Exercise lowers the risk of heart attack. It may, but to do so it has to be the right kind of exercise, which is to say, regular. If you sit at a desk all week and then go out and run two miles on Saturday or shovel out a whole driveway of snow, there's a good chance that the sudden exertion will trigger a heart attack.

But, if you exercise every day of your life, you can bring about certain specific changes in your body which will offer you a measure of insurance against heart attacks. For one thing, regular exercise appears to lower the level of cholesterol in the bood, thus preventing it from clogging arteries. Exercise also improves your lung capacity, bringing more oxygen into your body. It keeps your weight down and generally tones up your muscles, including, of course, the heart muscle.

eyebrows, eyelashes.

Once cut or shaved, eyelashes and eyebrows never grow back. It may seem like forever, but eyebrows and eyelashes do grow back. Eventually. The problem is that the tiny hairs in your eyebrows and eyelashes are not replaced on as regular a schedule as the hairs on your head or your body. The hair on your head, for example, is constantly falling out and being replaced with new hairs, so that except for situations in which great clumps of hair fall out you are not aware of the replacement. The eyebrows and eyelashes, however, grow on a different schedule: they grow for about ten weeks at a time and then stop growing for several months. As a result, a cut, shaved, or pulled-out eyelash or brow hair may not be replaced for as long as nine months.

eye color.

All babies have blue eyes at birth. The eyes of most

Caucasian babies do look blue at birth, even though they may eventually turn out to be green, hazel, or even dark brown. But the eyes of dark-skinned children, including Orientals, are brown right from the start.

Blue-eyed blondes are the most delicate of all people. There may be something to the folk tradition which, in Western civilization at least, always makes the tender heroine a blue-eyed maiden. In 1975, ophthalmologist Michel Millodot of the University of Wales Institute of Science and Technology studied the corneal sensitivity of 156 subjects (112 Caucasians, 12 Blacks, 15 Indians, and 17 Chinese).

His results showed that the corneas of brown-eyed nonwhites were about half as sensitive to pain as those of brown-eyed Caucasians, and only about one-fourth as sensitive as those of blue-eyed Caucasians. (Hazel- and green-eyed people fell somewhere in between.) If Millodot's findings are borne out, they would have fascinating implications. Differing corneal sensitivity, for example, might explain why some people have so much trouble accommodating themselves to contact lenses. It might mean that dark-eyed persons in general, and dark-eyed nonwhites in particular, would require less anesthesia and less medication for eye problems. And, perhaps most intriguing of all, if corneal sensitivity reflects overall body sensitivity, Millodot's study might explain why acupuncture has apparently been so successful among the dark-eyed Chinese.

eyes.

Reading in bed or in a moving car can ruin your eyes. None will do you any lasting harm, but each can strain your eye muscles, give you a headache or (in the case of reading in a moving car) make you sick to your stomach.

People who read in bed generally do so in positions which demand an almost impossible adjustment not from the eye or its lens but from the muscles which govern its movement. When these muscles are strained, they ache, just like any other muscles. Sit up straight in bed or in an ordinary chair, and there will be no strain on the muscles and no ache.

As for reading in a moving car, that also presents muscle problems, but is more likely to cause headaches and sometimes nausea as you try to watch a jumpy target. People who are subject to motion sickness know that concentrating on an immovable object, like the horizon, is one way to avoid a jumping stomach. But it is impossible to keep the page from moving in a car as you travel so that the letters you are trying to read keep moving. Watching them requires a constant readjustment of the eye muscles, which can produce strain, a headache, or sometimes nausea.

Cold water makes your eyes bright. A splash of cold water constricts the blood vessels in your eyes so that the surface of the eye looks clearer and, consequently, brighter.

Applying ice cubes to the eyes relieves fatigue. Cold compresses, yes (see above); ice cubes, no. The ice cubes can freeze the eyeball if left on too long.

See also SUNGLASSES.

F

※

---

face/facial expression.

    "Be careful, or your face will freeze like that." This is usually something a parent says to a kid who's got his face screwed up into some impossible expression, but actually it's better advice for an adult because our faces *do* "freeze" or wrinkle into the patterns of creases which we create whenever we smile, frown, talk, and so forth. There's absolutely no way to avoid wrinkles altogether, but it is true that smiling, which uses fewer muscles than frowning, builds up fewer wrinkle lines.

    People who live together eventually begin to look alike. Over the years, people who live together can begin, unconsciously, to mimic each other's facial and speech patterns and even to move in the same general way, so that while their original physical characteristics do not change, they begin to give the impression of looking like each other. In addition, researchers at the University of Alabama found, a few years ago, that people who live together long enough begin to develop a kind of internal resemblance, which is to say that their blood chemistries—the level of cholesterol in the blood, the amount of proteins, and so forth—come to be roughly similar.

fainting.

If you feel faint, put your head between your knees. Fainting is caused by a temporary rush of blood and oxygen away from the brain. Leaning your head down puts things back where they belong. However, when you feel faint, you also feel dizzy, and there is always the possibility that your body will simply follow your head down, which means that you can fall right off your chair. A much better idea is just to lie down flat on your back. The floor will do in an emergency.

A sip of whiskey will revive someone who has fainted. Never give a fainting person a sip of any liquid, since an unconscious person cannot control his throat muscles and may choke on the drink. A sip of whiskey is a particularly unhappy choice of liquid, too, because liquor lowers blood pressure, which makes it even harder for the blood to get back up into the brain.

Splashing water in his face will revive someone who has fainted. This mistakenly assumes that the "shock" of the water will revive the fainter. Unfortunately, the real shock may turn out to be the fact that the person who has fainted can choke on any liquid inhaled into the lungs through the nose or throat.

fasting.

Fasting shrinks the stomach. Could be. In experiments at the University of Texas Health Science Center in Houston, researchers discovered that rats that were deprived of food (fasting) or fed intravenously produced less gastrin, a gastrointestinal hormone necessary for the growth of the stomach and intestinal lining. As a result, the lining of both the stomach and intestines did shrink, or at least did not grow, according to Dr. Leonard R. Johnson, who conducted the experiments.

Fasting clears the head and cleans out the body. There's nothing surprising about the fact that the body, deprived of food, will eventually stop manufacturing solid waste, a condition some people consider "clean." Nor is there anything surprising about the feeling of light-headedness which accompanies a fast: the body, deprived of food, simply begins to cut down on the amount of oxygen it supplies to the brain. Less oxygen produces that light feeling in the head which sometimes leads to the hallucinations which fasters confuse with enlightenment.

Continued too long, however, fasting leads not to enlightenment but to death. The body, starved for food, begins to digest its own tissues and eventually loses the ability to process food entirely. At this point, there is no known medical treatment that can reverse the deadly process and the patient succumbs even if he finally consents to eat.

fat people.

Fat women are afraid of, or uninterested in sex. It sounds like a perfectly reasonable theory. In a society where fat is usually regarded as unattractive, a woman who allows heself to accumulate large amounts of fat could be suspected of hiding from or avoiding sexual encounters. But it now seems that this may be one of those cases where apparent logic runs head on into the results of scientific investigation, and loses.

Several years ago, researchers at the Michael Reese Hospital in Chicago interviewed sixty married women, thirty fat ones and thirty thin. Both groups reported approximately the same frequency of marital relations (about nine times a month), but the thin women said they were satisfied with that rate while all the fat women apparently wanted more. The researchers concluded that the fat women weren't eating to avoid sex but to satisfy a greater than normal appetite for food, which was probably matched by a greater than normal appetite for sex. To back that up, a psychologist at the University of Texas has reported that fat people seem to lack the ability to recognize satiation, in their appetite for food as well as for sex.

Fat people are jolly. Fat people are people and no more or less jolly than anyone else, although they may often assume a mask of jollity because society expects them to.

Fat people are warmer than thin people in the winter. It certainly seems logical to assume that layers of fat would keep one insulated against a winter's chill, but in this case logic is in disagreement with basic physiology. The nerve endings which allow us to feel heat or cold are right next to the surface of the skin, so fat people feel the chill the same way thin people do. However, while a thin person's innards can radiate heat quickly out to the skin, a fat person's fat can stop the radiating heat dead in its tracks, so that it takes longer than expected to get up to the skin's surface.

Fat babies are healthier than thin ones. It depends. In a society where food is scarce, a fat baby is obviously healthier than a skinny, starving one. But there is a wide difference between a child who is thin because of malnutrition and one who is lean because of proper diet. The healthy thin child looks like a miniature athlete, with bright eyes, good muscle tone, and quick, energetic movements. The starving child has dull eyes and dropping muscles and rarely moves about spontaneously. As for the fat child, in a society where enough food is available, the fat child is simply fat, and shows every indication of growing into a fat adult.

Some researchers have theorized, in fact, that feeding a baby enough to make it fat creates additional "fat cells" in the body which can never be eliminated. In adulthood, the individual faces the fact that his additional fat cells will swell with every bite and that, in order to be thin, he would have to live for the rest of his life on a diet which thin people would consider restrictive.

Children outgrow their "baby fat" naturally. This is rarely true. A child who is overweight and overfed into adolescence will almost always have weight problems as long as he lives. His extra fat cells make it impossible for him to be slim on a normal diet; if he wishes to lose weight and keep it off, he must expect to remain on a smaller than normal calorie allowance forever.

fear.

People can go white with fear. Faced with an immediate physical or emotional challenge, the human body responds with a series of instinctive reactions designed to prepare the body for the classic fight or flight. Among these responses is the constriction of surface blood vessels, which sends blood from the skin down into the muscles, where it helps to provide energy. When the vessels constrict, there is—temporarily—less blood flowing through them and the normal rosy or ruddy color of white or light skins disappears. At that particular moment, a light-skinned person may really look "white" with fear.

Animals can smell fear. Because they exist at a pre-language level, animals react to clues which we have come to call "body language." They also react to olfactory clues called phero-mones, chemical substances which animals release to signal sexual readiness or, perhaps, to warn an intruder away from a den.

There is little question that animals can use their instinctive understanding of body signals to "read" certain basic emotions, such as happiness, anger, and fear in human beings. In addition, frightened human beings often perspire heavily, and it is possible that there is an olfactory signal in the perspiration of fear which animals can recognize.

Even more interesting is the growing evidence that human beings also react to chemical signals, specifically, where sex is concerned. In 1971, for example, a study of a group of coeds at a suburban Boston college showed that, after a few months in a dormitory situation, the women's menstrual cycles began to synchronize. Six years later, researchers at San Francisco State University were able to synchronize menstrual cycles among young women volunteers by applying a bit of perspiration in alcohol to the volunteers' upper lips. The perspiration had come from a young woman with a history of "driving" someone else's menstrual cycle (that is, when she roomed with a friend, the friend's menstrual cycle began to synchronize with hers). A control group received an alcohol application with no perspiration in it. Among the women who received the "driver's" perspiration, menstrual cycles began to synchronize, ultimately coming within three days of the dominant woman's; among the control group, who did not receive the perspiration, no deviation from their ordinary cycles was noted.

In addition, researchers at the University of California in San Francisco have shown that volunteers can easily differentiate between samples of perspiration from men and from women, and babies have been shown to be able to recognize the scents of their own mothers.

Fear can make your hair stand on end. Sort of. When you are frightened, all your muscles tense, including the ones in your scalp. Tight scalp muscles can make the hair shaft stand up slightly. You'd have to have a real crew cut in order to get a true porcupine effect, but even long hair would ripple slightly if you were frightened enough.

"Scared to death." Severe emotional stress can produce bodily reactions leading to physical shock. First, there is a demand for adrenalin to constrict surface blood vessels, so that blood will be diverted deeper into the muscles, making them strong enough to allow a choice, "fight or flight." If the demand for adrenalin continues, and the blood vessels remain constricted, the entire body may eventually become starved for blood and, hence, for the oxygen which blood components carry. The result can be physical shock, a serious drop in blood pressure, which, unless relieved, can kill.

In so-called "civilized" countries, it is rare (or rarely admitted) that shock produced by emotional stress can kill. In more primitive societies, however, the witch doctor has always drawn his strength from his power to use suggestion to eliminate his enemies or to punish the wavering. The adrenalin shock produced by emotional stress is the "black magic" or "voodoo" which wipes out people who really believe that they are subject to a curse. The curse, of course, is of their own making.

fever.

Feed a cold and starve a fever. When you are running a fever, your body burns up energy faster than it normally would. The same thing happens when you get a cold, or, in fact, any other infection. The physiological rule of thumb, therefore, is that you would need more, not less, food when you have a fever.

However, people with fevers are miserable and uncomfortable. They have headaches and upset stomachs, may vomit, and, if the fever is high enough, may even be delirious. None of this is conducive to wolfing down a hearty meal, which is why folk wisdom counsels letting the patient take it easy for a few days, with liquids or, at most, a little boiled chicken or an egg. (In hospitals, where everyone knows that patients with serious fevers need food, intravenous feeding is the usual solution.)

Colds are supposed to be fed, but they pose other problems, namely that anything which disrupts one's sense of smell also throws off one's sense of taste. It is hard to eat when everything tastes like a variety of damp cotton. The usual folk remedy, chicken soup, has the advantage of being highly salted, sometimes enough to break through the tasteless, smell-less barrier of the cold. (NOTE: occasionally this maxim is reversed to read "Starve a cold and stuff a fever," which is still at least half wrong.)

You can "break" a high fever by making the victim sweat profusely. Perspiration is the body's normal response to an internal temperature heightened by infection or inflammation. The moisture has a cooling effect as it evaporates on the skin. It is for this reason that cooling-by-evaporation techniques such as forced persiration (piling blankets on top of a fevered patient) or alcohol rubs were so popular in the days before antibiotics or aspirin were available. Today, however, the drugs represent a much safer and more effective way to lower fever.

fever blisters. *See* COLD SORES.

fingernails.

Fingernails continue to grow after death. Alas for all the mystery writers who made a cracking good thing out of the coffin opened to show a corpse with two- or three-inch-long fingernails, the truth is that the nails do not grow after death, although the cuticle around them may shrink enough to make them look longer.

Fingernails grow faster in the summer than in the winter. The average growth of a hale and hearty finger- or toenail is about .1 millimeter every day. During the summer, this growth rate does speed up a bit. Nobody knows whether it is due to the warmth or the exposure to sunlight, with its increased dosages of vitamin D, or the fact that most of us seem to eat more healthful diets when we are out and running around in the summer.

Biting your nails will slow their growth. On the contrary, there is some evidence that biting the nails, like pruning a plant, can actually speed the rate of growth. However—and it's a big *however*—biting may shorten the nail's actual length from the cuticle to where it comes clear of the skin of your finger, so that if it is ever allowed to grow freely, it will not be as strong and flexible as it might have been otherwise.

Gelatin makes fingernails strong. There is absolutely no scientific proof whatsoever that gelatin (which is an inferior protein) has any specific effect on nail growth or strength.

"Bloodless," pale, or white skin under the nail indicates anemia. True. Extremely pale skin under the nails, as well as inside the eyelids or in the creases of the palm of the hand, may indicate anemia. (See SKIN COLOR.) On the other hand, tiny splotches of bright color under the nails, or nail hemorrhages, may be early symptoms of such diseases as scurvy, trichinosis, or liver disorders.

"Nail creams" can strengthen the nail. The nail itself, like the hair, is actually "dead" when it grows out of the cuticle. While creams may polish or shine this cornified layer of cells, nothing in the world is going to bring your nails back to glowing "life."

Nail polish "keeps the nail from breathing." Since the nail itself is already dead, the polish can't do anything to suffocate it. On the contrary, so long as you are not allergic to the polish (an allergy would usually show up in cracked or peeling nails or an inflammation of the skin around the nail) polish can protect the nail from the drying and cracking effects of air and especially dishwater. Polish remover can be drying, though, so most experts advocate touching up tiny chips rather than removing the polish and starting from scratch each time there is a chip.

Dark "moons" (or "blue" ones) in the nails of a seemingly white person indicate that there is some "black blood" in his background. This was once supposed to be a foolproof way to figure out if some apparently white person was actually a "quadroon" (a person with one black grandparent) or "octoroon" (a person with one black great grandparent) passing as a white. In truth, the skin color under the nails or on the palms of the hands simply mirrors that of the body in general. Light-skinned people have lighter palms and nails than dark-skinned people. Period.

fish.

Fish is brain food. In some specific instances, it can be. In landlocked areas, where the local vegetation is deficient in iodine (which is found abundantly in salt-water fish and in vegetables grown near the sea), iodine deficiency is possible. Without enough iodine in the body, the thyroid gland enlarges (goiter) and the production of thyroid hormones decreases. Since thyroid hormones are necessary to keep body and mine functioning at tiptop speed, people with iodine deficiency move and think more slowly than normal. If the deficiency is serious enough, people with normal intelligence may even appear to be retarded.

Today, iodized salt has pretty well eliminated the possibility of iodine deficiency in the United States, but when that was a real problem people usually found that eating fish made them feel better and also cleared up any mental fog. Hence, fish became "brain food."

Modern brain research has also shown another way in which fish (along with meat and eggs) may help stimulate the brain or at least transmit its messages to the body. All these foods are rich in lecithin, a major source of choline, which is, in turn, a chemical precursor of acetylcholine. Acetylcholine is one of many chemicals which act as transmitters for brain impulses within the body. Scientists have speculated that insufficient quantities of acetylcholine in the body may be responsible for mental problems, such as manic behavior, and for loss of memory.

fluoridation.

Fluoridated water causes cancer. Fluoridating various water systems and adding sodium fluoride to toothpastes, tooth powders, and dental sprays to prevent cavities have been standard practice for almost two decades now with no indication at all that they cause any ill effects in human beings. In addition, laboratory tests on mice, rats, dogs, rabbits, guinea pigs, and frogs have shown no incidence of cancer, tumors, or fetal defects traceable to the sodium fluoride. Moreover, since fluoridation can occur naturally, when drinking water flows through ground which is rich in fluorides (as in the American West), there has been ample opportunity to see exactly what long-term consumption of highly fluoridated water can do. The answer is that highly fluoridated water (naturally fluoridated water contains much more fluoridation than is normally added to water artificially) can stain teeth. And the fluorides do collect in the bones, making them heavier. But there is no sign at all that Westerners who have been drinking naturally fluoridated water all their lives have any more cancers or tumors than the rest of us.

food poisoning.

Food which smells good is safe. Not necessarily. Some forms of food poisoning, including (occasionally) botulism, may not always cause the food to smell bad. If you notice a can bulging at the ends, or if food just doesn't look right, throw it out. That's much safer than depending on your sense of smell, and much safer too than taking "just a taste" to test the quality. If the food has gone bad, that little taste can do you in.

Mold on cheese is safe. Mold growing on the outside of cheese can generally be scraped off and discarded, although some people may find this so unaesthetic that they throw the entire cheese out. Mold growing on the inside of the cheese, however, is another matter altogether. Interior molds are anerobic organisms, which grow in the absence of air, and they can be dangerous (botulism is caused by an anerobic organism). Wash your hands thoroughly after touching such a cheese, and wash down your counter, too. It's a good idea to wrap the offending cheese tightly in an airtight plastic bag. Then call the local Food and Drug Administration office, since FDA officials will be most interested in finding out exactly what was in your cheese. (Whenever you find suspicious foods, it is always a good idea to call the FDA; if the food is spoiled, they will issue a bulletin warning other consumers away from that particular batch of canned or packaged products.) NOTE: Interior molds which are meant to be there, such as the mold which makes blue cheeses "blue," are an obvious exception to this rule.

Canned tomatoes can't cause food poisoning. This rule is based upon the fact that *Clostridium botulinum,* the organism that causes botulism, cannot flourish in an acid medium. Since tomatoes (so long as they come from healthy vines and are sound, with no soft or decayed spots) are acid, they are safe from botulism contamination. For a time, it was believed that the newer varieties of "sweet," or less acid, tomatoes now popular in the United States were not acid enough to prevent the growth of the botulism organism. But, in 1977, studies at the University of Minnesota showed that there is really no such thing as a truly "low acid" tomato. The researchers studied 107 varieties of tomatoes, including some "sweet" ones, and found them all sufficiently acid to be safely canned in a water bath canner.

freckles.

Lemon juice, lemon juice and salt, buttermilk, or yogurt can bleach away freckles. Since each of these alleged freckle removers is acid and has a mild bleaching effect, each may produce a slight lightening. None, however, is a true freckle remover. Age, of course, may lighten freckles somewhat, as avoiding the sun will keep them from darkening. In any event, before attempting to lighten an individual freckle which seems to have gotten darker, it is always wise to check with your doctor so as to be certain that the "freckle" is not an incipient skin cancer.

fried foods.

Fried foods cause acne. No such correlation has ever been scientifically proven.

Fried foods cause cancer. Cooking oils, when heated excessively, degrade into substances which have been shown to be carcinogenic in animals. Never heat the oil until it smokes; never re-use cooking oils.

frogs.

Handling frogs causes warts. Yes, it can. So can using somebody else's damp towel or walking barefoot on a damp floor.

It works this way: warts are caused by viruses which flourish in damp or slimy places. A frog's skin certainly meets that criterion, so there is always the chance that the wart virus is living contentedly on the skin of that cute little frog you pick up out in the woods. If the virus is there, it can skip to your hand when you pick up the frog, and, if there is a crack in the skin on your hand, the virus can burrow in to cause the wart you caught by handling the frog.

Of course, the original association between warts and frogs had very little to do with a knowledge of viruses, since frogs were being blamed for warts as far back as Greek and Roman times when viruses were unknown. Probably the relationship was founded on the warty appearance of the amphibian's skin, which made it, rather than a fish or a swamp weed, the logical candidate to blame for warts which appeared on the hand of a kid who'd been playing around in the swamp.

frostbite.

Rub frostbitten areas with snow. Never. First, frostbitten parts of your body are *cold;* you want to warm them up, not chill them further. Second, the cells in the frostbitten skin are frozen and brittle. Rough treatment can only damage them further. To bring your frostbitten skin back to normal, plunge it into warm water (about body temperature; water that is too hot can burn skin which has no sensation and doesn't hurt when scalded). Then, gently massage the area so as to return circulation without injuring the skin. None of this will work on skin or fingers and toes which have already turned black; anything other than a tiny patch of whitened skin should get medical attention as soon as possible.

Give frostbite victims a nip of brandy. Medically, it makes sense. Frostbite occurs when the small blood vessels near the skin are so chilled that they go into spasm, interrupting blood flow to the affected area. Liquor is a vasodilator, which can sometimes help to alleviate spasming of the surface vessels so that circulation returns. The problem with liquor, of course, is that it often makes people careless. Too much, and one may forget the danger from the cold, which is why, after blizzards, alcoholics are often found frozen to death out of doors. Inside, however, near warmth, a nip or two can be a positive boon to the frostbite victim.

Stamping your feet can prevent frostbite. In general, anything that keeps your circulation going will prevent frostbite, and if your main problem is keeping warm while waiting for a bus, stamping your feet and moving about will certainly help. There are, however, limits to the cold which the human body can take, and stamping your feet is not going to protect you against frostbite in a truly Arctic or blizzard situation.

G

❖

---

garlic.

> **_Eating garlic (or hanging a bulb around your neck) protects you from germs._** The garlic plant (Latin name, _Allium sativum)_ contains two potent anti-bacterial principles, allicin (a recognized antibiotic) and alliin. Conceivably, generations of Italian mothers who fed their families garlic day after day may have been onto something, since it is at least theoretically possible that eating all that garlic would give you some of the antimicrobial properties of the plant. However, there is absolutely no indication at all that hanging a hunk of garlic around your neck will attract and kill germs the way flypaper attracts and kills flies. As the old joke goes, though, it could protect you from germs by keeping other people—and their colds— well out of catching range.

> **_Garlic stimulates digestion._** The essential oils in garlic can help relieve intestinal discomfort by expelling gas from the stomach and intestinal tract. Some people think of this as a digestive aid, but a lot more regard it as an embarrasssing nuisance.

Garlic is good for the heart. Like onions, garlic is a strongly-flavored food. In most folk wisdom, such foods are associated with strength; you have to be strong to eat them and once eaten they transfer their strength to the diner. More to the point, however, is the fact that in laboratory experiments, the essential oils in garlic, like the essential oils in onions, appear to have the ability to cut through and dissolve cholesterol. Whether or not this happens in the human body as well remains to be seen, but if it does, then garlic, like onions, really would be good for the heart.

See ONIONS.

german measles.

If a pregnant woman catches German measles, her baby will be deformed. During the first three months of its life, the embryo lacks the ability to recognize that the German measles virus is an "enemy," and cannot manufacture antibodies to destroy it. As a result, the virus which can be transmitted to the fetus through the mother's bloodstream continues to multiply and can cause such defects as deafness, cataracts, and heart malformations. Sometimes babies who pick up rubella (German measles) from their mothers are born with the live viruses still multiplying in their bodies.

The most dangerous period for the fetus comes during the first four weeks of pregnancy, when the possibility of the virus's damaging the baby is about 60 percent. The risk falls to about 35 percent during the second four weeks of pregnancy, and to about 7 percent in the four weeks after that.

As a result, women who have not had German measles, or rubella, as children are usually urged to be vaccinated before becoming pregnant. No woman should be vaccinated, however, unless she is certain that she is not pregnant, and no pregnancy should be allowed to begin until at least three months after the vaccination has been administered.

gin.

>**Gin with pepper in it is an aphrodisiac.** Pepper never dissolves in the intestinal tract, which means that it goes through the body as microscopic pebbles. As these tiny particles pass out through the urinary tract, they can cause an irritation which some people (masochists, to be certain) might regard as stimulating.

See also MARTINIS.

ginseng.

>**Ginseng increases potency and prevents aging.** Sorry, but there's no scientific proof at all to support the widely held belief that ginseng makes you potent and keeps you from the debilitations of age. Nor is ginseng an aphrodisiac, although it is interesting to speculate why it was thought to be.

Like the mandrake root, the ginseng can sometimes look a bit like the human body, with a long "trunk" and two "legs" branching off at the bottom. This faintly humanoid appearance made it easy to attribute medicinal properties to the plant, even though there was no scientific basis for them.

On the more positive side, ginseng does contain some B vitamins. And both Russian and Chinese scientists claim to have isolated substances in ginseng which influence cardio-vascular functions (though these conclusions have never been duplicated in the West).

glaucoma.

>**Glaucoma is a disease of advancing old age.** Generally it appears to be, but it may also be present (although rarely) in newborn infants.

>**Seeing halos around lights at night is a sure sign of glaucoma.** It is one of the symptoms. Others are redness in the eye, pain, and a blurring of vision, all of which can signal an elevation of

pressure within the eye which may destroy sight unless the process is halted (it cannot be reversed).

See also URINE.

gout.

     Women don't get gout. They do, but much less frequently than men do. The actual ratio is about twenty male victims for every woman with gout. And, since women usually do not develop the disease until after menopause, there seems to be a real basis for Hippocrates' assumption that gout is sex-related, which to Hippocrates meant that eunuchs did not get it and neither did young boys.

     Gout is a rich man's disease. Gout appears to be an inherited metabolic disorder which prevents the body from dealing correctly with purines, substances which are either taken in as food or manufactured inside the body. One by-product of purine metabolism is uric acid. Normally, the body excretes the uric acid it produces by metabolizing purines, but the gout sufferer seems unable to get rid of the uric acid in his blood. The uric acid collects and begins to break down into sodium urate, which then causes inflammation of the joints of the lower extremities, most characteristically, the big toe.

What has that got to do with rich men? Simple. Foods unusually rich in purines—sweetbreads and other organ meats and anchovies, for example—were ordinarily associated with the diet of the privileged classes. However, modern medicine has shown that a diet low in purines doesn't necessarily prevent attacks of gout, that a gout sufferer's own body may produce high amounts of purine even when the foods are "correct." Nowadays we know that people who get gout get it regardless of their economic status and sometimes regardless of their diets.

     Only intelligent people suffer from gout. It is true that there have been some spectacularly successful people on the historical list of gout victims: Alexander the Great, Charlemagne, Michelangelo, Luther, Calvin, and Charles Darwin. But there have been a lot of ordinary folk in there too, and there has never been any scientific correlation drawn between intelligence and gout.

However, modern research has shown that uric acid is similar to caffeine and other chemicals which can stimulate the cerebral cortex, so it is not impossible that a person who has an inherited inability to rid his body of excess uric acid might be receiving more mental stimulation than most people. So far, though, this one is still in the "fascinating but unproven" file.

Meadow saffron prevents gout. Meadow saffron, an herb which has been used ever since the time of the Greeks to alleviate the symptoms of gout, is the source of the modern drug *colchicine,* which can help ease the pain of a gout attack within hours and has been used, in small amounts on a daily basis, to prevent attacks before they occur.

H

✣

---

hair.

　　Shock can make your hair turn white overnight. Sort
of. Everyone loses some hair every day. The lost hair is gradually
replaced by new hair and is almost never noticed. Severe emotional or
physical trauma, though, may interfere with this normal schedule of
loss and replacement. Either more hair than normal may fall out, or it
may take longer for new hair to grow in, or, if the shock is severe
enough, the first new hair which grows in may not be as darkly
pigmented as one's original hair. In any case, the hair, though it won't
go white overnight, will look a little lighter for a while.

　　On the other hand, people suffering from *alopecia areata* (reversible
patchy baldness) or *alopecia totalis* (reversible total baldness) often
tend to lose only pigmented hair. The hair which remains is grey or
whitish and so may look as though it had turned white very quickly, if
not overnight. A new treatment developed at the University of
Alabama shows promise in dealing with these two kinds of baldness.
Dr. Leopoldo F. Montez has treated alopecia patients with a drug
called halcinonide, often used to treat eczema and psoriasis, and he
reports that patients taking halcinonide showed a new growth of hair

within a few months. (The drug definitely does not work with true male pattern baldness.)

See also FINGERNAILS.

Brush your hair one hundred times a night to make it shine. Brushing the hair does make it shinier because it stimulates the oil glands in the scalp. But brushing also can split and pull out hair, causing those two banes of the beauty-parlor set—split, frizzy ends and thinning hair. A much safer course is to message the scalp. You get the same stimulation of the oil glands without damaging the hair.

A natural-bristle brush is safer than a nylon one. It depends on the brush. Some nylon bristles are sharp and can cut or split the hair, but there are nylon bristles whose ends are rounded and will not damage the hair.

Hair grows faster in the summer. Yes, hair (again, like fingernails) grows faster in warmer weather. It also grows faster when you are young than when you are old.

Washing your hair every day will make it fall out. Like your face and your hands, your hair gets dirty every day and washing it will only make it clean. It can be damaging, however, to comb, pull or brush wet hair. When it is wet, your hair loses its natural elasticity, and even ordinary pressure may break or pull it out. Let your hair dry slightly before setting it to avoid this extra breakage. (A slight hair loss every day of your life is normal.)

Cutting your hair frequently makes it grow. It's not exactly like pruning a tree, since cutting off the end of a strand of hair won't cause it to sprout branches. Frequent trimming, however, is still a good idea because it gets rid of the (invariably) splitting ends and gives you a sleeker, shinier look.

Singeing the hair "seals in its nutrients." Your hair is hollow, but it is also made up of dead cells. There is nothing inside to seal in, and singeing the ends only splits them.

hands, cold.

Cold hands, warm heart. This is not the sort of thing you can put your money on, if what you mean by "warm" is "passionate," but the maxim does have a sort of logic to it. Women in the childbearing years, when most courting is done, are generally at least mildly anemic, and anemic people do often have cold hands. So a cold hand doesn't necessarily mean that the lady herself is cold, and advising young lovers that "cold hands" mean "warm heart" at least gets the ball rolling. In point of fact, of course, your heart is warm (pumping blood) as long as you are alive, no matter how icy your hands.

hangovers.

The best cure: "the hair of the dog that bit you." While fads such as oxygen, tomato juice, raw eggs, or various antacids have come and gone, dedicated drinkers have always maintained that the only real cure was the "hair of the dog." Now it seems that there may be some evidence to show that, while it won't cure a hangover (only time does that), a little nip may have some beneficial effects.

Sheboygan, Wisconsin, doctor James R. Hoon is a gastric specialist particularly adept at using a gastrocamera, which allows him to take pictures of the inside of the stomach by inserting a flexible tube through the mouth and down the throat. While using his camera to photograph the effects of various drugs, Dr. Hoon got the chance to photograph the stomach of a hangover victim before and after that legendary morning-after nip. The camera showed that alcohol did, indeed, quiet the jittery stomach of the hangover victim—almost certainly, according to the Center of Alcohol Studies at Rutgers University, because it is a tranquilizer which acts as a central-nervous-system depressant and calms jumpy nerves.

However, too much of a nip can put enough alcohol back into your bloodstream to trip you off into another hangover, so this is a cure to be wary of.

(Raw eggs) (tomato juice) (milk) cures a hangover. If you are hungry, the food may make you feel better, but the tremors and nausea of a hangover really only go away with time. Much better to avoid them entirely by watching your drinking the night before.

Bourbon gives you a worse hangover than vodka. It may. Some alcoholic beverages (bourbon, blended whiskeys, rum, and brandy) contain high concentrations of flavoring agents called *congeners,* and these ingredients appear to be implicated as causes of the pain and much of the misery of the hangover. Gin and vodka have almost none of these congeners, and appear to be less likely to cause the headaches normally associated with the morning after. In one experiment conducted by a researcher at Davis Medical School at the University of California, young adult volunteers were fed either bourbon or vodka in a party setting complete with dancing and merrymaking. Afterward, bourbon drinkers outnumbered vodka drinkers as hangover victims by a margin of approximately ten to one.

Aspirin cures a hangover. It may relieve the symptoms, but nothing except time (which gets the alcohol out of your body) can really cure a hangover.

hats.

Wearing a hat prevents colds. Alas, nothing but avoiding cold viruses (or staying strong enough to resist those you run into) can prevent a cold, but wearing a hat when it's cold outside can have a significant effect on how cold you feel. The blood vessels in your scalp don't constrict as efficiently as those near the surface of your arm, for example, or your leg. When those blood vessels constrict, they send significant amounts of blood down into the muscles where it remains warmer than it would up near the surface of the skin. But very little blood is sent away from the vessels on the surface of the scalp. Most of the blood there is chilled before it circulates back into your body to chill your muscles and inner organs. How serious is this kind of chilling? Researchers have estimated that going without a hat can cut the effectiveness of your body's ability to heat itself by as much as 50 percent.

heart, broken.

She died of a "broken heart." The phenomenon of people dying soon after the death of a husband, wife, sweetheart, child or close friend is well known, but has always been more or less ascribed either to chance or to some vague romantic impulse. Recently, however, a team of researchers in Sydney, Australia, has come up with evidence to show that the death from a "broken heart" is really one more solid example of the effects of stress on the human body. The researchers set up a study involving twenty-six persons whose husband or wife had died recently. The results of the study, reported in *Lancet,* the British medical journal, showed that all the subjects evinced suppression of various aspects of their immune systems (the systems which protect the body from infection and disease), as well as an alteration in hormone levels. Quite simply, the researchers concluded, the stress of grief affects some persons so strongly that it makes them more susceptible to death not from a heart which never physically "breaks" but from the results of actual physical malfunction.

heart disease.

Women don't have heart attacks. Yes, they do, but at a much lower rate than men. About ten years ago, the rate of heart attacks in the 35-to-45-year-old groups was 57 per 100,000 women *vs.* 300 per 100,000 men; the rate for both groups has been dropping since then. As yet, no one has been able to pin this drop on anything specific, although there is a lot of evidence that a major change in the American diet, with less emphasis on red meat and saturated fats, may be at least partially responsible.

See also BRANDY, CHOLESTEROL, GARLIC, ONIONS, SEXUAL INTERCOURSE, VITAMIN E.

heat prostration.

People suffering from "heat prostration" should be immersed in an ice-water bath. Although they are usually grouped together under the catchall term of "heat prostration," there are really two different kinds of problems connected with severe overheating and/or overexertion. The first, which is known technically as heat exhaustion, is a weakness which follows excessive perspiration (which causes an excessive loss of water and salt). Heat exhaustion can be quickly relieved by feeding the victim liquids and some salt (potato chips, for example) or ideally a liquid, such as fruit juice, which has some salt in it. The second form of heat prostration, heat stroke, is more serious. It involves an upset of the body's thermoregulatory system, resulting from extreme overexertion, or in some cases from circulatory impairment due either to old age or to some illness. When this system shuts down, perspiration stops. The body cannot be cooled, temperature soars (sometimes to as high as 105 or 107 degrees) and the victim feels dizzy, weak, and nauseated. Sometimes, he may faint. The most important thing to do is to lower the body temperature, and this was once thought to be accomplished best by plunging the victim into an ice bath. Today, however, we know that the sudden shock may be dangerous for the victim's heart; modern emergency treatment for heat shock involves the application of cold, wet sheets as dressings, plus the restoration of fluids to the body.

In hot weather, everyone needs salt tablets. Unless you work in front of a blast furnace, casually swallowing salt tablets may do your kidneys more harm than it does your body good. In normal circumstances, simply eating salty foods, like potato chips, and drinking adequate amounts of fluids will keep your salt/water balance in safe bounds.

height.

Every generation of Americans is taller than the one before. A delightful fact of American history, much beloved by the

makers of American movies who, right up through the 1950s, made a
virtual visual cliche out of the (short) immigrant father and his (tall)
American son. What lay behind the cliche was quite simple, of course.
Until the middle of the fifties, every succeeding generation of Ameri-
can children got a better and more balanced diet than the generation
before. The result was, naturally, taller, bigger, stronger people.
When the American diet more or less stabilized a few years after the
Second World War, so did the growth rate. American children born to
American-born parents aren't really noticeably taller any more.
(Immigrant parents, however, may still find themselves producing
taller children. And that holds for countries other than America, too.
In Israel, for example, where a major part of the population is
immigrant, the nutritionally spurred growth of the next generation is
an exuberant fact of national life.)

hemophilia.

Hemophiliacs can bleed to death from a pinprick.
Hemophiliacs lack or are deficient in the clotting factor which allows
blood to clot or form a scab quickly if the skin is broken. It's true that
massive injury will produce massive loss of blood and that even a
pinprick will ooze longer on a hemophiliac's hand than it would on a
normal hand. But, a truly minor injury can be clotted by applying
immediate pressure, so pinpricks are not really all that dramatic, even
to a hemophiliac.

The real problem that the hemophiliac faces on a daily basis is
uncontrolled internal bleeding; under the skin or into a joint. Minor
injuries which would produce only minor bruises in non-hemophiliacs
can produce large, swollen blood clots under the skin of hemophiliacs.
Worse, repeated uncontrolled bleeding into a joint can, in time,
destroy the joint and cripple the patient.

Hemophilia is a royal disease. Hemophilia is a genetic
disease, carried in the X chromosome. Women have two X chromosomes; men have an X chromosome and a Y chromosome. Therefore,
a woman may have a defective X chromosome and a normal one and,
since hemophilia is a recessive trait, the normal X chromosome will

dominate and the woman will be apparently normal. (It is theoretically possible, but rare beyond any odds, for a woman to inherit two defective X chromosomes and, thus, hemophilia.) However, if she has a male child, and passes her damaged X chromosome on to him, his other sex chromosome, the Y, will not be able to counter the hemophilia gene and he will be a hemophiliac.

The idea that this kind of heredity is somehow royal lies in the fact that so many of the prominent and therefore visible victims of hemophilia were members of the ruling houses of Europe during the nineteenth century. In truth, virtually all of the royal hemophiliacs could trace their disease back to a single source, Queen Victoria. The Queen is now believed to have harbored a mutated gene (there had never been any hemophilia in her family before her) which she passed on to some of her sons and daughters. As they married, intermarried, and ascended to the various thrones of Europe, hemophilia made its way through the ranks of their children. The most famous of its victims, of course, was Alexis, the son of Nicholas, the last Czar of Russia. Nicholas' wife, Alix (later Alexandra) was a granddaughter of Queen Victoria. Some people have even speculated that Alexis' hemophilia was a contributing factor to the Russian Revolution and the overthrow of the Czar, for the child's suffering made his mother a willing disciple of Rasputin (whose presence was often said to have calmed Alexis and eased his incidents of bleeding). Rasputin, in turn, was one of those who urged that the Czar refuse to compromise with the Russian reformers, a decision that spurred on the forces of the revolution.

Royals and revolutions aside, however, hemophilia is a distressingly democratic affliction, which strikes wherever the genetic predisposition exists.

hiccups.

Swallowing air, drinking ice water, eating very hot foods, or talking while eating can cause hiccups. Absolutely. So can anything else which abnormally stimulates the phrenic nerve, which controls your diaphragm, or the vagus nerve, which controls the glottis or opening from your mouth into your throat. Ordinarily, these nerves trigger a spasm only when necessary to protect you. For example, if you start to swallow a large chunk of food or an unexpectedly large amount of liquid, the glottis will clench to keep the food or liquid from falling into your windpipe, and the diaphragm will clench in an involuntary upward movement to force the invading food or liquid out of your throat. Once the danger is past, the glottis and diaphragm will relax. If they do not, they may continue to spasm in the characteristic gulping pattern we call hiccups, and this pattern may be triggered by something as seemingly innocuous as a surprised, gulping intake of air.

Simply holding your breath can cure an attack of hiccups. It may. What you are trying to do is interrupt the spasm reflex which has taken control of the vagus and phrenic nerves. Holding your breath can increase the amount of carbon dioxide in your lungs and blood, which will stimulate your brain to send a signal to the diaphragm, which begins to deepen its contractions so as to bring oxygen into the body. The hope is that these deepening contractions will break the pattern of the shallower, hiccupping contractions.

Breathing the air from a paper bag cures hiccups. It may, for the same reason that holding your breath may be able to end an attack (see above).

A cold compress or a cold knife on the back of the neck can cure hiccups. The phrenic nerve, one of those involved in the involuntary spasms of the hiccup reflex, runs up the back of the neck. Theoretically, at least, chilling the nerve may trip the pattern of involuntary spasms, ending the hiccups.

Drink a glass of ice water to cure hiccups. If you can get the water down, it can chill the vagus nerve, which controls the spasming of the glottis and may end the hiccups.

A sharp yank on the tongue can cure hiccups. This is another way to add stimulation to the vagus nerve at the back of the mouth and possibly end its spasmodic contractions.

Sneezing cures hiccups. Sneezing causes contractions in the muscles near and around the glottis. This contraction just might interrupt the spasmodic contractions of the vagus or phrenic nerves and, therefore, stop the hiccups. Alas, it's not easy to trigger a sneeze just exactly when you want to. Sniffing at some pepper usually does it, though, which is why sniffing pepper has also occasionally been touted as a folk remedy for hiccups.

Hiccups are a minor problem. In most cases, hiccups are a minor annoyance. Obviously, if yours stop when you sneeze or inhale the air from a paper bag, then you've got nothing to worry about. But sometimes hiccups can be so serious as to constitute a life-threatening situation—that is, an attack that continues hour after hour for several days can eventually interfere not only with eating and sleeping but with breathing as well.

Treatment for this sort of attack may involve one of three things, each of which is, essentially, a stepped-up version of the folk or home remedies for minor hiccups. First, doctors may attempt to stop nerve and muscle spasms with drugs, just as you might try to quiet them with cold. The commonest drugs used for this purpose are anti-spasmodics and central-nervous-system depressants, such as the barbiturates. Second, the medical people may use what is really a very sophisticated version of the "breathe-the-air-from-a-paper-bag" technique, substituting a machine which delivers oxygen plus carbon dioxide for the paper bag. The last remedy on the list is the most drastic: surgery to cut the phrenic nerve and paralyze the diaphragm, ending its spasms.

homosexuals.

Homosexuals can't have children. Some homosexuals may be sterile and some lesbians barren, but that's an individual condition and has nothing whatsoever to do with sexual preferences. Most homosexuals are just as capable as most heterosexuals of having as many children as they wish.

I

✳

---

ice cream.

Ice cream has enough food value to serve as a substitute for milk. It's true that ice cream, which is made from milk, has all the nutrients in it that you'd expect to find in the milk. But that doesn't mean that you can substitute one cup of ice cream for one cup of milk and come up equal, nutritionally speaking. First of all, there will be a lot more calories in the ice cream, about 255 in a cup compared to 160 in a cup of whole milk or 90 in a cup of skim milk. Either kind of milk will give you about 9 grams of protein per cup, while the ice cream will offer only 6. And when it comes to calcium, the main mineral you want from milk and milk foods, there are about 288 milligrams in a cup of whole milk, 296 in a cup of skim milk (skim milk has less milkfat and more milk solids than whole milk) vs. 194 milligrams of calcium in a cup of ice cream.

Of course your ice cream does have more of some things than milk does. Fat, for instance. There are 14 grams of fat in a cup of ice cream as against 9 grams of fat in a cup of whole milk and a skinny little trace of fat in the skim milk. And, there are about 8 grams of saturated fats in that cup of ice cream; only 5 grams in the whole milk and, once again, just a trace in the skim milk. All that fat, of course, is why ice cream does, admittedly, have more Vitamin A than either whole or skim milk: 590 I.U. in the ice cream, 350 I.U. in the whole milk and a measly 10 I.U. in the skim milk.

See also ICE WATER.

ice water.

Ice water gives you headaches. Not just ice water, but also ice cream, ice cream sodas, sherbet and all kinds of chilled or chilly dessert delights can trigger sudden headaches. What happens is that the cold food stimulates the nerves which run from the top of your mouth (your palate) straight up into the brain. To end the headache, you have to warm and soothe the nerves, and, according to a serious report published in the prestigious *New England Journal of Medicine,* you can cure your cold-caused headache by curling your tongue back so that it presses up against the top of your mouth, warming the palate.

Ice water makes you cough. This works on the same principle as the headaches, except that the ice water is triggering different nerves. In addition, some people have a kind of allergic reaction to very cold food, drink or weather and may cough or sneeze or their eyes may tear whenever they run into one or another of these chilly stimuli.

See also BUTTER, EXERCISE, EYES, SPRAINS

impotence.

Masturbation makes you impotent. There is absolutely no physiological reason at all for masturbation to have any effect on a man's ability to attain and maintain an erection and then to ejaculate upon orgasm. However, there are a lot of emotional strings attached to masturbation, and many people feel guilty about the act. Since a man who feels guilty, frightened or remorseful is often unable to perform sexually, you might just say that this is one instance in which thinking makes it so.

See also SEXUAL INTERCOURSE, SEXUAL POTENCY.

infertility.

A man who is infertile doesn't produce any sperm at all. Not so. An infertile man usually produces sperm, but either he doesn't produce enough, or they are not sufficiently motile to impregnate his partner. In some instances, therefore, artificial insemination which makes things easier for the sperm by delivering them right up where they are needed may do the trick by giving the sperm the headstart they needed.

See also HOMOSEXUALITY, MASTURBATION, SEXUAL INTERCOURSE, SEXUAL POTENCY.

insecticides.

Insecticides cause cancer. There is no general rule to this one. Some insecticides and some herbicides (chemicals which destroy vegetation and are usually used in battle to wipe out the enemy's natural jungle cover) may be carcinogenic, but the chemicals have to be evaluated one by one to be sure. Agent Orange, for example, the chemical herbicide widely used in Viet Nam, now appears to have been carcinogenic, but DDT, the most famous insecticide, has never been shown to cause either cancer or tumors in laboratory animals despite its widely-accepted reputation as a potent carcinogen.

iodine.

Painting a cut or scrape with iodine makes it sterile. Hardly. A swipe with the iodine applicator may wipe out a few bacteria in the general area, but the skin's own natural bacteria will move right in again. However, the iodine can be strong enough to injure sensitive tissues around the wound and do more damage than good. The best treatment for superficial injuries is probably just to wash out the dirt and debris with plain soap and running water. It's clean and it's soothing and, best of all, it doesn't even sting.

Rubbing iodine and baby oil on your skin before going out in the sun guarantees a good tan. No way. The iodine may stain your skin a pleasant tannish brown, but it won't do a thing to protect you against the sun's burning rays. Neither will the baby oil. Most baby oil is simply plain mineral oil (read the label), and mineral oil, like vegetable oils, is simply unable to keep your skin from burning in the sun. Use this combination and you'll end up not with a tan but with a burn. And probably a bad one, at that, since the illusion of protection may convince you to stay out in the sun longer than you ordinarily would

See also FISH.

IQ.

A child's IQ is a good indicator of how well he will do later in life. A child's IQ may give a fair idea of what his IQ will be when he grows up, but it is a poor indicator of how he will perform. According to research done by Robert B. McCall at the Fels Research Institute in Yellow Springs, Ohio, you have about an 80 percent chance of predicting performance in adult life from a child's IQ at 13 years of age, but that drops back to about a 60 percent chance at age 18. The correlation between IQ at age 7, when the child is in second grade, and his later performance is also about 60 percent, which is really not good enough to make firm decisions about education. Yet many schools base their evaluation of children on IQ at just this age, and therefore many children are shortchanged insofar as expectations about their abilities are concerned.

IQ never changes. External conditions, such as family environment, not to mention diet, can affect a child's IQ severely (or well) enough to raise or lower it more than ten points, and sometimes twenty. And just growing up can change a person's IQ as experiences in the outside world (outside school and home, that is) have their effect. IQ, in other words, is not a measurement that remains constant through life.

See also FISH, TWINS.

iron deficiency anemia.

See POTS AND PANS.

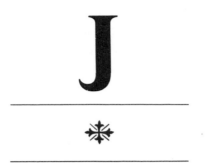

jade.

Closing the body orifices with pieces of jade keeps a corpse from decaying. The jade has no effect at all on the body, which turns to dust as all corpses must. But, as bacteria destroy the proteins of the body, an ammonia-like liquid is produced and this makes hash of the jade, turning it to a white, chalky substance.

K

kissing.

    Kissing spreads germs. Any disease that can be handed on through an exchange of bacteria or viruses in the saliva certainly can be exchanged with a kiss. Mononucleosis spreads this way; so does a cold, the flu, and a host of other undesirables, including venereal diseases, which can be spread through kissing if there are active sores on the lips or if there is oral/genital contact.

L

lemon juice.

Lemon-juice rinses make the hair shine. Because lemon juice is an acid, it can, in specific situations, add a shine to your hair. First, if you wash with a soap or alkaline shampoo, even repeated rinsings with clear water will leave a skim of alkali (which used to be called a "dulling soap film") on your hair. The acid in the lemon juice will dissolve and remove this skim, returning the shine to your hair. However, since most modern shampoos are made of detergents or synthetic cleansers, which are either acid or at least not alkaline, this is an old-fashioned procedure that's really not necessary.

However, lemon juice's acid can deal with purely physical dulling of the hair, too. The outer part of the hair shaft is covered with tiny, scalelike formations called *imbrecations.* When you wash your hair, these small scales are ruffled and stand up every which way. When that happens, the light which hits your hair is deflected in dozens of directions, so that it does not shine back evenly and your hair looks dull. Anything that helps smooth the imbrecations back into place helps to create a smooth surface on the hair shaft, which reflects light evenly and looks, naturally, shiny. An acid like lemon juice can cause the imbrecations to lie down flat and thus the hair to look shiny.

Lemon-juice rinses lighten the hair. The citric acid in lemon juice is a (very) mild bleach and may, if you put it on and then go out in the sun, lighten blond hair slightly.

Lemon juice (or the inside of the lemon rind) can lighten skin. The citric acid in the juice or rind can lighten freckles and blemishes on the skin—but very slightly, and only temporarily.

Lemon juice (or the inside of the lemon rind) can soften skin. In addition to its slight bleaching effect, the citric acid in the lemon juice or rind also has a slight keratolytic effect—that is, it can help dry and flake off the top layer of the dead cells on the skin, thus making the skin itself look smoother and possibly paler.

Drinking lemon juice and hot water every morning encourages regularity. There are several possible reasons why this may be true:

First, the acidity of lemon juice and water can stimulate the secretion of gastric juices, giving one a definite feeling that something is going on in the area of the stomach and colon.

Second, research into the causes of obesity seems to show that falling body and skin temperatures are often interpreted by the brain as a signal that it is time to eat. Individuals differ, but body temperature is likely to be low as you get out of bed; it rises as you begin to move around. Therefore, a steaming cup of lemon juice and water, or even a mildly hot one, can raise your internal temperature, making you feel more fit, (that is, less "hungry") and ready to begin the day. In short, it acts as a tonic.

Finally, as serious dieters have always known, quantities of liquids can sometimes fool the body into thinking that they are quantities of food. Your stomach can feel full on a glass of water, and certainly a cupful of lemon juice and water would do nicely. Feeling that it has been handed something bulky, the stomach and intestinal tract may be tricked into going on to the next step, which is getting rid of the waste material. Ergo, lemon juice and hot water may act as a mild laxative.

It is only fair, of course, to point out that almost any warm breakfast can accomplish all the things we have just attributed to a time-honored, but rather unpalatable, folk remedy.

A drop of lemon juice in the eyes makes them bright. Only with tears. This is an old European "beauty trick," and a perfect illustration of the maxim that women have to suffer for beauty.

licorice.

Licorice aids digestion. The root of the licorice plant, glycyrrhiza, has been a part of the folk-medicine arsenal since the time of the Greeks, who used it as a digestive, a laxative, and, of course, a flavoring. Its most important medical use, however, was not confirmed until late in the 1960s, when it was discovered that one of the substances in the root, carbenoxolone, protects the lining of the stomach against erosion by stomach acid. Carbenoxolone, and several other drugs extracted from the licorice plant, are now used to help ulcers heal. Licorice itself, in the form of syrup of glycyrrhiza, is used to flavor medical extracts and syrups.

Licorice is a reducing agent. A "licorice diet," like a grapefruit diet or any one of several dozen other fad diets, can have potentially serious consequences. In the case of licorice, the problem is potassium depletion, since licorice contains the salt of an acid which causes the body to excrete potassium at a higher than normal rate. The symptoms of potassium deficiency (which has been suspected to be the cause of deaths associated with a liquid-protein regimen) are muscle weakness and generalized malaise. In some cases, it has caused death. (Note: Licorice candy made with artificial licorice flavoring won't produce any of these effects, of course, but it won't make you skinny, either.)

lightning.

You can be electrocuted by touching someone who has been struck by lightning. People who have been struck by lightning may be burned, but their bodies do not contain stored currents of electricity, and you may touch them without fear for your own safety. There are, however, instances in which persons who have been electrocuted accidentally can be dangerous to others. If the electrocuted person still is in contact with a live wire, for example, he can transmit its current to anyone who touches him. Or, if a person has been electrocuted by stepping into water—a swimming pool, perhaps—in which there is live current from an exposed wire, anyone who wades in to rescue him may also be electrocuted.

People who have been killed by lightning can come back to life. Many life processes, including respiration and heartbeat, are triggered by electrical impulses within the body. Being struck by lightning interrupts the body's own electrical system, which means that breathing and heartbeat may cease. Prompt mouth-to-mouth resuscitation and heart massage, the same treatment used in cases of cardiac arrest due to a heart attack, may enable the body to start going again, thus bringing the lightning-struck person "back to life." That is why, if you see a group of people hit by lightning, you should always head for the ones who look dead. Any who are breathing or moving on their own will almost certainly recover spontaneously.

liquor.

Liquor makes you sexy. True, it does lower inhibitions, but it also lowers physical effectiveness, and many a would-be seducer has found himself in embarrassing straits after matching his date drink for drink.

Men hold their liquor better than women do. The human body is mostly water, but the exact percentage depends on whether the body in question is male (60 to 70 percent water) or female (50 to 60 percent water). The extra liquid in a man's tissues dilutes alcohol faster than a woman's body does, and, since straight liquor is more intoxicating than diluted liquor, a man does show less effects from the same amount of alcohol. In other words, although individual tolerances may vary considerably, a man who drinks two ounces of whiskey will generally be less affected by it than a woman who consumes the same amount.

"In vino veritas." Too much liquor often lowers the psychological barriers which usually keep us discreet, or at least polite. Having drunk too much, a lot of us turn pugnacious, loquacious or just plain teary, and end up saying things we would never have said while sober. Whether or not these things we say are true is another question entirely.

Never mix whiskey and wine in one night. Actually, you can even mix the two in one cocktail (a Manhattan is whiskey plus a wine, vermouth) and still come out all right. The real point is that too much of both will do you in, and if by mixing whiskey and wine you mean two Scotches and a couple of glasses of wine, the answer is obvious: Don't. (Of course exact amounts depend on the individual's level of tolerance for alcohol.)

Whiskey and water is a milder drink than whiskey and soda. Water dilutes the alcohol and slows its absorption. Soda dilutes the alcohol, but carries it past the stomach to the small intestine faster, and since alcohol is absorbed into the bloodstream from there, you will indeed feel the effects of a Scotch and soda more quickly.

Drinking makes people wittier. No. But it's all a matter of perception. Alcohol dulls the senses so that the drinker tends to talk faster and louder, but that doesn't make him wittier, only more noisy. It may also make him ruder, for, as a study undertaken by three researchers at the University of California at Irvine showed, people who have had a few belts often forget to listen—or actually just don't hear—when other people talk. They interrupt when others are talking and generally make nuisances of themselves.

Liquor has only "empty" calories. It depends. Nutrients from corn, barley and such are lost in the distilling which gives us whiskies, gin and vodka. But wines are not distilled. They are fermented from fruit juices and may contain nutrients from the juices. In fact, California doctor Salvatore Lucia, co-author of *The Wine Diet Cookbook,* says a glass of wine has significant B vitamins and minerals, along with anywhere from 95 to 178 calories, depending on the wine. (There are about 150 calories in 1 oz. of 100 proof whiskey.)

American Indians couldn't handle the white man's firewater. In 1971, this myth got a big boost from a Canadian study which suggested that Canadian Indians and Eskimos metabolized alcohol at a slower rate than Canadian whites. If that were true, it would mean that the Indians would show the effects of the same amount of alcohol faster than the whites.

But there were two catches in the study. First, the Indians were hospitalized patients, while the whites were healthy individuals. Second, the metabolism of alcohol was measured simply by Breatholizer, an inexact determination of metabolism rate at best. Which is why it is even more interesting to note the results of a 1976 study by Dr. Lynn J. Bennion of the National Institute for Arthritis, Metabolism and Digestive Diseases and Dr. Tingkai Li of the Indiana University School of Medicine.

This study, which compared alcohol-metabolism rates of healthy Indians and healthy whites, gave the firewater myth a severe drenching, for it showed that, if anything, the Indians metabolized liquor faster than the whites. One reason: American Indians tend to be heavier than whites of the same height and build, and heavier people metabolize liquor faster. (The metabolism rates were determined by having each group swallow a 50 percent ethyl-alcohol solution on an empty stomach. In addition, the researchers measured liquor metabolism in the liver tissues of seven Indians and seven whites who were undergoing routine liver biopsies for Hodgkin's disease. The second group showed the same differences in the ability to metabolize liquor.)

No matter how much you drink, it won't affect your liver so long as you eat a decent diet. Cirrhosis of the liver has always been assumed to be caused by a combination of overindulgence in alcoholic beverages and a lack of necessary nutrients. Now two researchers at Mount Sinai Hospital in New York have been able to show that the cirrhosis is a direct result of the toxicity of alcoholic beverages and has nothing whatsoever to do with the drinker's diet.

In the experiment, Drs. Emanuel Rubin and Charles Lieber fed a liquid diet to two groups of baboons. (Baboons were chosen because their life span is fifteen years, long enough to see the cumulative effects of overindulgence in liquor.) The only difference in the diets was that one included alcohol, equivalent to a fifth of whiskey each day, while the other did not. Both diets had exactly the same amounts of vitamins, minerals, and other nutrients. At periods starting with nine months and extending up to four years, the duration of the study, the baboons fed the alcohol began to develop the symptoms of cirrhosis, fatty liver, and hepatitis, all attributable to alcohol abuse.

See also ALCOHOLISM, BRANDY, CHAMPAGNE, COLOR BLINDNESS, GIN, HANGOVERS, MARTINIS.

M

✤

---

mandrake root.

The mandrake is an aphrodisiac. Because its form is faintly humanoid, with branched "legs" descending from a straight "trunk," the mandrake root has often been credited with human reactions or with the ability to influence human activities. One old myth, for example, says that the root screams when it is pulled from the ground. Another insists that the mandrake is an aphrodisiac. Neither myth is true, although, like some other reputed aphrodisiacs (pepper, for example, or cantharides), the dried and powdered mandrake is quite caustic and may irritate the urinary tract.

marijuana.

Marijuana increases sexual potency. No way; although smoking marijuana may produce a feeling of relaxation and pleasure, it can actively interfere with the male body's ability both to produce sperm cells and to produce and/or sustain an erection.

According to research done by Dr. Robert Kolodny at the Reproductive Biology Research Foundation in St. Louis, heavy use of marijuana (which is defined as approximately five marijuana cigarettes a day) will, after four weeks, produce a significant drop in the production of the bodily substances which help produce the male hormone, testosterone. After the fifth week the body's testosterone level drops, and after another three weeks, the body's production of sperm cells begins to fall. By the end of two months, the testosterone level may have dropped by as much as one-third, which means that libido (the desire for sex) practically disappears. Happily, the whole process can be reversed if the use of marijuana stops.

Obviously, few people smoke five marijuana cigarettes a day on a continuing basis, but it may take less than that to produce some sexual problems. Researchers from Walter Reed Army Medical Center in Washington, D.C., and the University of Massachusetts at Worcester, gave laboratory rats small doses of Delta nine tetrahydrocannabinol, the ingredient in marijuana which produces the "high" associated with the drug. The rats were given the drugs during the forty days of their life which correspond to adolescence in human beings and, as a result, the rats (which developed normally otherwise) had smaller-than-normal testicles, and some of them were unable to produce sperm cells at all. It is not inconceivable, therefore, that while adults would have to overindulge in the drugs for long periods of time before it adversely affected their libidos or sperm production, adolescents might run into trouble much more quickly with much lower doses.

Smoking marijuana is just a step on the way to stronger drugs. Despite the propaganda to the contrary, people who smoke marijuana almost always stay with it, preferring its relatively mild high to the dramatic and sometimes deadly kicks of more potent drugs. The single exception to this general rule occurred during 1969, when the Nixon adminstration was pushing "Operation Intercept," an attempt to shut off the delivery of marijuana from Mexico. Operation Intercept created a marijuana famine in this country, during which thousands of young people first tried stronger stuff, such as barbiturates and LSD. One can only speculate that had marijuana remained relatively easy to obtain these youngsters would never have had the need or desire to move on to other drugs.

martinis.

Martinis pack more of a punch than other alcoholic beverages. An ordinary drink usually consists of about an ounce of liquor, straight or in combination with maybe three to eight ounces of a mixer. Since the high you get from alcohol is less if (1) the alcohol is diluted in water or mixer, or (2) the time between drinks is stretched out, you can easily see how one Scotch (one ounce) or one Scotch and water (one ounce of Scotch plus three ounces of water) is a lot less likely to make you tiddly than a Martini, served in a glass which contains two or three ounces of plain gin flavored with a dash or even just a hint of vermouth. Now if you were to dilute the Martini by serving it on the rocks, you would slow its punch somewhat, but there is still no way to alibi away the difference between three ounces of gin and one ounce of Scotch. (By the way, Martinis made with vodka would follow exactly the same rules.) And there's one more thing. Some people are allergic to the herbs and botanicals used to flavor gin, and some people are allergic to gin in combination with shellfish.

masturbation.

Masturbation causes insanity or blindness or makes hair grow on the palms of your hands. Ridiculous. However—and it is a big "however"—if you believe that these things are true, then it is always possible that your own sense of guilt about masturbating can cause any and all of the marvelously imaginative punishments which men and women can inflict upon themselves. That includes rashes, hives, nervousness, and, if things are carried to extremes, impotence. (No matter how guilty you feel, however, hair will *never* grow on the palms of your hands because the skin there, like that on the soles of your feet, has no hair follicles.) The cause in all cases, however, is the guilt, not the masturbation.

Masturbation makes you sterile. When men ejaculate, they release a fluid which contains sperm cells. Frequent ejaculation, whether through masturbation or intercourse, can lower the number of sperm cells present in the ejaculate, although it will not interfere with potency (the ability to achieve an erection and ejaculation). Simply refraining from masturbation or intercourse for a day or two will allow the body to bring the sperm count back up to normal.

Masturbation is "self-abuse." On the contrary, it can be a kindness during periods when ordinary sexual contacts are not available, for adolescents, say, or for adults who are forced, at any stage of their lives, to spend long periods of time alone or separated from their partners. For infants and growing children, masturbation is simply a natural part of the process of discovering their bodies.

maturation.

Each new generation of women matures earlier. According to a study of female puberty conducted jointly by the National Institutes of Health, the Massachusetts Institute of Technology and Massachusetts General Hospital, middle-class girls in America reach puberty at exactly the same age now as their mothers did, more than thirty years ago. Individual ages at menarche (the first menstrual period) can vary widely, of course, from as early as nine years to as late as seventeen. But the results of the puberty study (which was released in 1976) show that on the average the age at menarche was exactly the same in 1943, 1954, and 1973: 12.8 years.

(NOTE: It is true that among some groups of females the age at menarche has advanced with later generations. This sort of change is attributable to a more nutritious diet. Poor diet can retard maturation; a good diet can bring it within "normal" age limits, which may, in some cases, seem to produce menarche at an earlier age.)

Girls mature earlier in tropical climates. Actually, extreme climates whether hot or cold tend to slow down maturation, not speed it up. In fact, virtually every objective scientific study on this subject has shown that girls in temperate zones mature up to a year or so earlier than girls in tropical or Arctic climates.

So the myth of the tropical child-woman, which was given so much weight by the experiences of American and European missionaries and sailors who explored and settled the South Pacific during the eighteenth and nineteenth centuries, really rests not on physical facts but on differences in cultural orientation. First, women in the tropics may have looked younger to Western eyes than did women in temperate zones. Second, sexual behavior among tropical societies was usually far less restrictive than that accepted as normal by Europeans and Americans.

As a result, when one of these sailors or missionaries ran into a childlike, sexually active woman, he simply assumed that she was more mature at an earlier age than the women he had left at home, when the truth was that she was almost certainly a sixteen- or seventeen-year-old acting on the demands of a physical maturity which the ladies at home put into cold storage until it was "proper" to exercise it (that is, with marriage, which in Western societies has rarely been intelligently linked up with the onset of physical maturity).

meat tenderizers.

"Tenderized" meat will eat away your stomach walls. The reasoning here is that anything which is strong enough to soften up raw meat is strong enough to do serious damage to your stomach. However, the "tenderizing" element in meat tenderizers is an enzyme, commonly papain, which comes from the papaya plant, and it is inactivated once heated. So, while the papain can indeed break down the fibers of the meat, once you cook the meat, its power to break down muscle tissue ceases.

medication.

The latest medicine is the most effective. On the contrary, a 1977 report released by the World Health Organization pointed out that all the world's health needs could be adequately served by 210 essential drugs. The committee which compiled the report went on to stress the fact that the tremendous increase in the numbers of new drugs put on the market each year did not correlate with an increase in health. Quite aside from that, it is important to note that the newer a drug is, the less information there will be about its possible side effects and adverse reactions, not to mention its value. That's not to say that spectacular discoveries about remedies for exotic or simply endemic diseases should be ignored; but in the general run of things, proven drugs are better than unproven ones.

menopause.

Women who have gone through menopause can still sometimes get pregnant. Usually, the onset of menopause is a gradual event. A woman may miss a few menstrual periods and then, sporadically, begin to menstruate again before stopping entirely. For this reason, doctors always advise women who do not wish to become pregnant to continue to use contraception for at least one full year after their last menstrual period. Women who have gone through a full year without menstruating are, in all normal circumstances, considered to be past the possibility of becoming pregnant again.

There is no longer any need for sex after menopause. There is exactly as much "need" for sex after menopause as there was before, although women who did not enjoy intercourse before menopause often use its onset as a reason to avoid sex entirely. It is true that shrinkage of vaginal tissue may make intercourse slightly more uncomfortable, but with sufficient artificial lubrication there should be no serious discomfort, and many women, no longer having to worry about the possibility of pregnancy, actually find sex after menopause much more enjoyable.

Menopause causes cancer. Obviously, this is generally taken to mean that menopause causes cancer of the uterus, a form of disease which is much more prevalent in women who have gone through menopause than in women who have not.

It is possible that the shift in hormonal balance which comes with menopause, when a woman's supply of estrogen diminishes, may be linked to the rise in uterine cancers after menopause. But it is also important to understand that simply living longer makes it more likely that one will develop some form of cancer, since cancer is primarily a disease of older age.

As for the benefits or risks of administering estrogen to post-menopausal women, the picture is simply unclear. At first, it seemed that giving estrogen to these women increased their chances of developing uterine cancer. But, in 1978, a study at Yale University appeared to show that there was no correlation at all between the administration of estrogen after menopause and the chances of developing uterine cancers.

Menopause makes you fat. It will if you expect it to and begin to eat accordingly, but millions of women have sailed through menopause with their dress sizes intact.

Menopause cures migraines. Curiously, migraine sufferers do often find that their headaches lessen or go away entirely when menopause begins. Whether this is due to a physical or a psychological change has never been scientifically divined.

menstruation.

Young women become fertile as soon as they begin to menstruate. Sometimes, but not always. In some instances, there may be a gap as long as two years between the time a girl begins to menstruate and the time she is able to conceive. (To be practical about it, though, women who do not wish to become pregnant should begin using contraceptive devices as soon as they become sexually active.)

You can't get pregnant during a menstrual period. Women ovulate approximately fourteen days before menstrual bleeding begins; the egg remains in the uterus for as long as forty-eight hours. Since sperm entering the vaginal canal before ovulation can live for as long as two or three days, a woman is presumed to be fertile two days before and two days after ovulation. Now, if the menstrual cycles are regularly twenty-four or more days long, the five-or six-day menstrual period can be a "safe" time. However, if the cycles are very short or so irregular that some menstrual periods are only fifteen to nineteen days apart, a woman may already be ovulating during the last day of her menstrual period, which means it would be "unsafe" for her to have unprotected intercourse at this time. (NOTE: The length of a menstrual cycle is measured by counting from the *first* day of bleeding, not from the *last*.)

You can only get pregnant during your menstrual period. There are a lot of women who, because they do not understand the physiology of the menstrual cycle, think that the uterus is always filled with blood, which does not escape because the mouth of the uterus, the cervix, is closed tight during most of the month. Comes the menstrual period, the cervix supposedly opens so that the blood can spill out. Using this logic, one might assume that at this point sperm could enter the uterus and fertilize an egg. Thus, to avoid pregnancy, one would only have to avoid intercourse during the menstrual period. Of course, this is wholly counter to the truth, which is that (1) the uterus is never "full of blood"; the lining simply builds up each month in preparation for pregnancy and sloughs off when none occurs; (2) the cervix never opens and shuts to allow or prevent the flow of blood or sperm; and (3) the fertile period of the month comes during ovulation, which is roughly fourteen days before menstrual bleeding.

During her period, a woman performs badly on any kind of test, physical or intellectual. For years, many women have accepted without question the belief that their ability to do well in school or on the athletic field varied with the phases of their menstrual cycles, with the lowest point coming right before the monthly period. In addition, there have been a number of attempts to bolster this belief with scientific evidence, showing that the rising and falling levels of hormones in a woman's body during any given month would affect her athletic or intellectual capacity.

However, all these theories and this belief have one thing in common: they are based upon the women's own reports of their increased or decreased ability to compete in school or in athletics. The conclusions about the disruptive effects of "premenstrual tension," for example, are drawn from reports in which women said it happened. But objective tests of performance show quite another story. In Olympic competitions, year after year, women have won gold, silver, and bronze medals with no regard at all for the phases of their personal cycles. In one notable example, an American woman swimmer took three gold medals and broke a world's record while competing at the height of her menstrual period.

The truth, according to a recent study reported in *Science* magazine by Diane N. Ruble of Princeton University, seems to be that even though many women believe that they are less competent during their periods or right before, most objective measurements of their performance show that there is no real difference at all which can be tied to the phases of the menstrual cycle. Ruble's subjects were forty-four women undergraduates at Princeton University. For purposes of the study, each subject was told, arbitrarily, that she was either premenstrual or in the middle of her cycle. And, no matter what the actual state of her body was, each woman began to behave as she expected she would according to the condition which Ruble had told her she was in. "Premenstrual" women, for example, began to report changes in eating habits (many women gain weight right before their periods) water retention, and general discomfort. "Intermenstrual" women, who might, in truth, really be premenstrual, reported none of these symptoms.

Women gain weight right before their periods. They may or they may not. It depends upon whether or not they change their eating habits so as to increase the calories they consume (see above). Sometimes bloating or swelling of tissue (a temporary condition) is mistaken for weight gain.

Menstrual cramps are really "all in your head." Sometimes yes, sometimes no. Although emotional factors may cause some women to exaggerate the normal discomfort of uterine contractions during a menstrual period, there are real, physical reasons that explain why others experience more pain than normal. For example, endometriosis (the implantation and growth of uterine tissue in places other than the uterus) can cause pain not only during menstruation, but during intercourse as well. So can pelvic inflammatory disease, or PID, a group of infections affecting the uterus, the ovaries, or the Fallopian tubes.

In addition, women who have heavy clotting during the menstrual period also experience pain and cramping. A study at Cornell Medical Center in New York City suggests that the cause of the clotting in an over-production of prostaglandins (hormones) in the uterus and suggests, also, that taking aspirin the day before the bleeding begins can alleviate the pain since aspirin has anti-clotting abilities and can keep blood clots from forming in the first place.

Menstruation cleans out the "bad blood." There is absolutely no difference at all between menstrual blood and the rest of the blood in the body. As a matter of fact, the loss of blood during the menstrual period is now generally regarded as the explanation for the difference between male and female hemoglobin counts, and the consequent widespread mild anemia among women of childbearing age. At one time, a hemoglobin count of about 11.5 was regarded as "normal" for women, while the "normal" count for men was something on the order of 13.5. (A hemoglobin count indicates the percentage of red blood cells in the blood. Since red blood cells carry oxygen, a lack of them can leave you feeling weak and tired.) However, before menarche and after menopause, female hemoglobins are right up there on the "male" level. During childbearing years, when a woman is menstruating, iron supplements are commonly used to raise the hemoglobin count and cure mild anemias.

The touch of a menstruating woman can turn milk (or wine) sour. Surely this one sounds like the quintessential old wives' tale, with more than a little prejudice against women thrown in besides. But the straight fact is that, in societies where the sanitation is dismal, this is possible and probable. And not only during menstruation.

The bacteria which ferment milk (and wine) are usually of the genus *lactobacillus*. One variety of lactobacillus, *L. bulgaricus*, teams up with another organism, *Streptococcus thermophilus*, to turn milk sour but palatable; what the two bacteria produce is, of course, yogurt.

Now for the connection between menstruating women and lactobacillus: the organism lives in the mouth, and outer genital area. Therefore, a woman who touched this area and then milk (a sequence not unlikely during menstruation in a society where sanitation is primitive) would be likely to transmit some bacteria, and the bacteria would, without doubt, turn the milk or wine sour.

A menstruating woman should never pick up a newborn baby as it will suffer from cramps if she does. The same old story with the same tenuous possibility of its being true. If the woman's hands are dirty and she transfers bacteria from the vaginal or anal area, it is not inconceivable that the child might catch some bug that could cause stomach upset and cramps. Obvious solution: wash your hands before picking up the baby.

It is dangerous to bathe or swim during the menstrual period. Although it may be unaesthetic to swim in a public pool unless a tampon is used to stanch the menstrual flow, neither bathtubs nor swimming pools pose any real danger to a menstruating woman. In fact, both may be positively beneficial, since the exercise of swimming and the warmth of a medium-hot bath can relax knotted muscles sometimes responsible for menstrual cramps.

The myth is so persistent, however, and so widespread that it is interesting to try to pin down the roots from which it sprang. There are three possibilities: (1) the belief that, during menstruation, the uterus is open and vulnerable to invading substances, like water; (2) the fear that hot baths will make the menstrual flow so heavy that it will result in anemia; and (3) the fear that chilling can be dangerous during the period.

Obviously, the first is false. The uterus does not "open" during the period and, while water may flow in and out of the vagina during a bath or swim, only liquids under pressure could be forced past the vagina, through the cervix and up into the uterus. As for reason number two, it is true that a very hot bath may increase the menstrual flow slightly, but never enough to cause serious anemia.

Which brings us to the third possible reason for avoiding baths and swimming pools. In 1977, two researchers at Michigan State University, Dr. Loudell F. Snow and Dr. Shirley M. Johnson, interviewed forty Michigan women to find out how knowledgeable they were about menstruation and the female reproductive cycle. The interviews turned up an amazing store of medical old wives' tales. Among the most common was the idea that becoming chilled while menstruating could either stop the flow of menstrual blood or cause tuberculosis. (This last was most common among Southern women, black and white alike. Latin America women carried the idea of chilling one step further, believing that eating cold foods could be fatal. In this case, "cold" referred not to temperature of the food, but to the composition. Fruits, for example, are considered "cold" foods, as are vegetables.)

Sometimes, the fear of chilling keeps menstruating women not only from bathing and swimming, but from going out into the rain, as well.

If you catch a chill while menstruating, bleeding will cease. (See above.)

A chill during menstruation can cause tuberculosis. (See above.)

Menstruating women should not go out of the house on a rainy day. (See above.)

Never eat citrus fruits or other acid foods while menstruating. This idea has great currency among many Southern women, black and white alike, who believe that acid foods will dry up the menstrual flow, with death a certain result. Actually, the only likely result is that these women will, for a few days at least, be living on a diet deficient in Vitamin C.

A woman can't get a good haircut while she is menstruating. In a society which prohibits bathing during the menstrual period, a woman is unlikely to wash her hair and it would begin to look dirty and lanky. Such hair isn't just unappealing; it lies flat or sometimes crimped on the head and cannot be cut well, even by a skilled hair stylist. Clean hair, however, behaves exactly the same way during the period as it does at any other time of the monthly cycle.

It is worth noting that this myth may sometimes be restated to read, "A woman *shouldn't* get her hair cut while she is menstruating." In that case, it takes on a different meaning. In primitive societies, the fear of allowing an enemy to have any piece of oneself—a small snip of hair, a fingernail paring—is great, for the piece of oneself is the same as oneself and allows one's enemies to work black magic. Where that kind of belief is prevalent, it would obviously make sense to keep anyone from collecting a lock of hair from a woman who is presumed to be at her "weakest" (during menstruation). But in twentieth-century America it makes no nevermind, at all.

migraine headaches.

People who suffer from migraine headaches are more intelligent than other people. In his book *Headaches* (Doubleday), Dr. Arthur S. Freese describes a study of more than nine thousand schoolchildren in which the results showed that there was no significant difference at all in intelligence between the kids who got migraine headaches and those who didn't. Actually, the single most striking characteristic that migraine sufferers seem to share is perfectionism, not necessarily intelligence.

Women get migraine headaches more often than men do. If you go by how often each sex is likely to ask a doctor for help in combatting the pain of migraines, this is absolutely true: more women than men (by a ratio of about ten to one) complain about migraines. However, there is always the possibility that men simply do not seek treatment for migraines. When a man asks for help with headaches, it is usually for "cluster" headaches—that is, severe and sometimes devastating headaches which occur in clusters, four or five a day, say, and then may disappear for weeks or months or years at a time.

Migraine headaches are allergic reactions. Sometimes they are. The most common allergic triggers for migraines seem to be chocolate and tuna fish.

See also MENOPAUSE, VINEGAR.

milk.

Milk is the "perfect food." The origins of this belief are perfectly obvious: babies do well on their own mothers' milk and many babies are able to take in milk from cows or goats with little or no trouble. Then, too, adults with digestive ills have often been given milk as a soothing food and seemed to do well on it. But, for millions of people, including such non-Caucasians as many Chinese and Japanese and most of the Blacks in this country, milk is far from perfect. In fact, they cannot digest it at all. Their bodies lack the intestinal enzyme *lactase,* which breaks down the *lactose,* or sugar, in milk. Without lactase, the milk sugar cannot be digested and instead it ferments in the stomach, causing cramps, gas, diarrhea, and other intestinal ills.

There is some speculation that lactase deficiency is one reason for the popularity of yogurt among non-Caucasian populations in the Middle East, since yogurt is, in effect, predigested milk, whose sugars have been broken down by bacterial action. In recent years, there has been research done (notably at the University of Rhode Island) on the practicality of producing "predigested milk," that is, milk to which lactase has been added. Of course, that wouldn't help people with milk allergies, nor would it do away with the fact that milk can often exacerbate the results of other allergies simply because drinking a lot of milk or eating a lot of milk products can produce mucus in air passages.

Finally, even if you don't have any of these problems, you should know that milk is deficient in adequate amounts of a number of nutrients (iron, for example), and that while it may very well be a super addition to your diet, it is far from being the perfect food.

Adults don't need milk. The human body needs calcium as long as it is alive, and, while some people (children as well as adults) cannot tolerate milk, those who can will find it, by far, the most economical source of calcium. If you want to avoid the cholesterol, or butterfat, in milk, you have only to switch to nonfat milk or to instant dry nonfat milk, which has more protein and calcium per ounce than ordinary liquid milk; you can add solids to as much or as little liquid as you like. (You can even enrich liquid nonfat milk with a spoonful of the dry milk. The result is a low-fat but richer-tasting beverage.)

Warm milk before bedtime can help you get to sleep. Yes, it may. Cool, warm, or hot, milk contains tryptophan, an amino acid which appears to have definite sedative effects.

Line your stomach with milk before an evening out and you won't get drunk. It's good advice, although you would do just as well to eat a thick steak, a cheese sandwich, or any other high-protein meal. What you are doing isn't actually lining your stomach, in the sense of painting the walls with some kind of barrier. You are putting protein in there so that it will slow down the absorption of the alcohol you drink. And the slower the absorption, the less likely you are to feel any untoward effects of a reasonable night's indulgence.

miscarriage.

Jumping up and down, or falling, can cause a miscarriage. If the pregnancy is a normal one and the fetus is developing as it should, it is highly unlikely that this kind of physical activity will shake the baby loose from its mother's womb. Pregnant women, after all, have been known to walk away from automobile or even airplane accidents with their pregnancies uninterrupted. The fetus which is aborted spontaneously after physical exertion is often discovered to have been defective in some way. The miscarriage would almost certainly have happened even if the mother had lain flat on her back in bed for nine months, because nature often terminates pregnancies which are not proceeding normally.

In addition, the newest line of research shows that some mothers' bodies treat the growing fetuses as invaders. Their immune systems reject the babies as surely as their bodies would reject the transplant of kidneys or blood transfusions when the types did not match. Women who abort spontaneously for this reason may be helped by drugs which suppress the action of their immune systems, but such treatment is experimental at this time.

A severe emotional shock can cause a miscarriage. The same rules apply here as above. Miscarriages which follow a severe emotional shock are usually coincidental and probably would have occurred even if the shock had not.

See also COTTONWOOD; BATHS, HOT; ROSEMARY.

moon.

A full moon drives men mad. People have always recognized a certain connection between the phases of the moon and human behavior. The legend of the werewolf, or man who turns into a wolf at the full moon, is the most dramatic rendition of this folk wisdom, but there are more gentle reminders, such as the fact that the word "lunatic" comes from *luna,* the Latin name for the moon.

Now it may not be true that a full moon drives men mad, but it certainly does seem to make them do some very strange things. Police records, for example, have always shown an increase in violent crime as the new moon appears, and in 1972 Dr. Arnold L. Lieber of the University of Miami made it official. Dr. Lieber put together a chart which showed all the homicides in Miami for a fifteen-year period arranged according to the phases of the moon. The chart clearly showed that the murder rate went up about a day before the new moon, reached a peak when the moon was full, and then began to decline, only to repeat the entire cycle with the next rising of the new moon. In Philadelphia, a similar study of admissions to psychiatric wards showed them rising as the moon did.

While we now have the data to show the possible truth in this maxim, we don't yet have the medical explanation. It would seem logical, however, that the gravitational pull of the moon, which influences all the tides on earth, may in some way affect the liquid balance in our bodies so as to influence our moods.

See also THUNDERSTORMS; WEATHER.

mud.

Mud (or manure) takes the sting out of insect bites. The old wives who invented this one knew that a damp, cool dressing can make itchy skin feel better. Since insect bites and bee stings are most likely to happen out in fields or pastures where there is a lot of mud and manure around, those seemed to be just the dressings needed. What the old wives didn't know is that either of these remedies carries the possibility of infection or, worse, tetanus. Bites and stings are puncture wounds, and something you pick up from the ground in an open field is almost certain to carry tetanus spores with it. Tetanus spores in a puncture would spell obvious trouble, which is why doctors recommend that you stick to water dressings for the itch and antihistamines or desensitizing shots for the allergic reactions. (In cases of potentially severe allergic reaction, your doctor may even want you to carry an emergency kit with you, one that contains a hypodermic of adrenalin.)

Mud makes a super facial. As it dries on your skin, mud hardens and "tightens," pulling impurities to the surface. In addition, when you wash it off, you also wash off the top layer of dead cells, so that the skin looks softer and smoother. That's the theory, and it works best with mud made from earth which is rich in *clay,* the base for some of the commercial face masks sold today in cosmetics departments. (Other masks are made of synthetic substances or various gums which also dry and tighten, pulling impurities to the surface and removing the top layer of cells.)

mushrooms.

Poisonous mushrooms blacken silver spoons. It is not inconceivable that there may have been a chemical reaction between one particular mushroom and one particular silver spoon (or maybe the spoon was just tarnished to begin with), but, according to the Brooklyn Botanic Garden, that has nothing whatsoever to do with the safety of the mushroom, and there is no truth at all to this myth. To be safe, avoid all wild mushrooms unless you are expert at differentiating them. Even then, it's not a bad idea to stick to commercially grown fungi.

Mushrooms which do not kill immediately aren't dangerous. A belief in this myth is said to have done Claudius Caesar in. Like any good emperor, he had his food tasted in advance. If the taster died, Claudius declined the dish. But the mushrooms whipped up for him by his wife Agrippina and his stepson Nero were slow-acting. Both Claudius and the taster expired, a little later than expected, but dead as doornails, nonetheless. Again, your best bet is the mushrooms you buy at the supermarket.

N

✤

---

natural foods.

     Foods grown in rich soil have more vitamins than foods grown in poor soil. The "richness" of the soil, which is to say, its mineral content, has absolutely nothing to do with the amount of vitamins in fruits and vegetables, since vitamins are manufactured inside the plant itself. A mineral-rich soil, however, can increase the mineral content of certain foods.

     Foods grown with organic fertilizer are more healthful than those grown with chemical fertilizer. As far as a plant is concerned, it doesn't matter a whit whether the fertilizer it is fed starts out as organic (that is, made from living matter, such as manure) or "chemical," since the plant cannot use the organic fertilizer until it is broken down by bacteria into its inorganic or chemical components. The inorganic components, or minerals, derived from chemical fertilizers are exactly the same, chemically speaking, as those derived from organic fertilizers.

     Natural foods are better for your skin. It depends. Obviously, such natural foods as fruits and vegetables are good for any body, but if your natural diet is high in kelp, sea salt, saltwater fish or shellfish, spinach, peanuts, wheat germ, or gluten bread, you may find that you are going to have a lot of trouble with your skin. The reason is very simple, of course. The first seven items on the list are high in iodine, and the last two (and shellfish) are high in androgens; both substances may cause an outbreak of acne or pustular eruptions on even the smoothest of complexions.

newborn babies.

You have to slap a newborn baby to make it take the first, vital breath. Babies born to mothers who have not had anesthesia usually breathe fairly easily, but if the mother was anesthetized, the baby will be too, and some shock is necessary to make it breathe. Because the child is slippery, a doctor often grabs it by the heels and holds it up for a slap on the rump. According to Dr. Edmund S. Crelin of Yale Medical School, however, that grip can be dangerous, for it may dislocate the baby's hips. In some cases, the doctor says, it has even crippled newborn children for life. A much safer procedure, in Dr. Crelin's view, is cradling the child and dipping it into a bath of cool water, which is just as successful—and a much less traumatic way—of helping the infant to take its first healthy gasp of air.

A baby born with bumps on the head is a "child of the devil." Occasionally, babies are injured during birth so that a cephalo-hematoma, or small collection of blood, forms between the bone of the skull and the membrane over it. As this injury heals naturally, it may become filled with a calcium deposit, a small hard bump once known as "devil's horns." The calcium will eventually be reabsorbed into the body and the bumps will disappear. Of course they have no connection with anything even remotely supernatural.

Never bathe a newborn until the cord falls off. The water could run into his body and drown him. Actually, it's a good idea to keep the stump of the cord clean, for the encrusted blood is an ideal place for bacteria to take up residence. In washing the baby, there is absolutely no chance at all that you can allow water to run into his body through the "belly button."

Very bright lights will damage a baby's eyes. Babies are just like adults in this regard: the only light that will cause permanent damage to our eyes is the light of the sun, which, if it is allowed to shine directly into the eye, can burn blind spots into the retina, or a "sun lamp," which can do the same thing. Most of us, babies and adults alike, blink our eyes or turn away from the sun instinctively, to avoid this kind of damage. As for ordinary bright incandescent lights, like those used to take pictures of the newborn child, they can be temporarily annoying, but won't cause any lasting problems.

See also CAUL, EYE COLOR.

nosebleeds.

Tilt your head back to stop a nosebleed. The practical reason for accepting this folk remedy is obvious: tilting your head back does stop the blood from dripping out of your nose. However, if it doesn't drip out, it will run into your throat (where it might cause choking) or into your stomach (where it could cause nausea and vomiting). So overcome your instincts and tilt you head slightly forward to get rid of the excess blood. At the same time, pinch the bridge or the tip of the nose shut so that a clot will form inside and stop the bleeding. In some cases, it may be necessary to have a doctor pack the nose with gauze in order to get a sufficiently firm clot to form.

Put a piece of ice or a cold knife on the back of the neck to stop a nosebleed. The physiological justification for this old wives' tale is the fact that the large blood vessels which feed blood to the nose run up the side and back of the neck. Chilling blood vessels causes them to contract, so presumably chilling these would cut off the supply of blood to the nose and thus end the nosebleed. In practice, of course, you would need an unbearable amount of chilling to cut off the flow of blood through major veins and arteries. If you really want to use cold compresses, the place to apply them is on the side of the nose, where you may affect the small blood vessel inside which is actually bleeding. However, pressure is much more likely to do the job quickly, which is why pressure on the bridge or side of the nose is the standard treatment for a minor nosebleed.

People with a tendency to nosebleeds should avoid heights. True. The question is, how high is high?

To figure that out, you have to understand the simple physiology and physics involved. Fact number one: as you go higher, the air pressure drops; the higher you go, the lower the pressure of the air is. Fact number two: the pressure inside your veins and arteries (your blood pressure) stays essentially the same. When you reach a height at which the pressure inside your blood vessels is significantly higher than the air pressure outside, the possibility exists that blood in your veins and arteries will begin to seep through the vessel walls, pushed through by the higher pressure inside.

Some people with fragile blood-vessel walls and very high blood pressure can begin to experience this effect at surprisingly low heights, sometimes as low as the seventh, eighth, or ninth floor of an ordinary office building or apartment house. Others with strong blood vessel walls and very low blood pressure might be able to climb several thousand feet up the side of a mountain without any untoward bleeding. People with frequent nosebleeds, however, obviously aren't in the latter class, and heights that lower the outside air pressure precipitously may well trigger a nosebleed for them. Only experience can show you exactly where your particular high is.

People with a tendency to nosebleeds shouldn't fly in airplanes. There is a noticeable difference in cabin pressure between unpressurized planes (like a small one-engine job or a small helicopter) and a pressurized plane like a 747. But, no matter what plane you get into, you will notice some variations. If you are going to have problems with nosebleeds, they will almost certainly come on takeoff, when the pressure inside the cabin is lower than the pressure inside your body. Whether or not one particular person will have a problem depends, once again, on the individual blood-vessel wall strength and blood pressure. People with ear problems will also notice the ups and downs of airplane cabin pressure, but, unfortunately, none of the remedies which work for ears can be adapted to strengthen the blood vessels inside the nose.

See also CHEWING GUM

O

onions.

Onions are good for the heart. Onions are sharp and pungent, and you have to be "strong" to eat them so some people reason that they must be good for your heart, making you strong as the sharpest onion. There may however, be more going for the onion than a simple belief in sympathetic medicine. Researchers in India have reported the results of studies at the Department of Cardiology at the R.N.T. Medical College in Udaipur which clearly show that the essential oils of both onions and garlic help to reduce the level of cholesterol in the blood. Perhaps the lowly onion and garlic bulbs may come to serve as cheap and effective aids in reducing the buildup of waxy deposits in blood vessels, which appears to be implicated in most deaths from "heart attacks."

operations (surgical).

"It's just a minor operation." Although some surgical procedures are clearly more difficult than others, there is no such thing as a truly minor operation. The administration of general anesthesia always carries with it the possibility of cardiac arrest, brain damage, postoperative pneumonia, and lengthened recovery time. In addition, when scalpels are in evidence, the possibility of hemorrhage is always present. Even so routine a procedure as a tonsillectomy is responsible for approximately three hundred surgical deaths each year. All of this explains why whatever surgery is done should be absolutely necessary.

orgasm.

    See CONTRACEPTION, VIRGINS.

oysters.

    Never eat oysters in months without an "r." It does make some sense, even though the wonders of modern refrigeration makes it possible to keep oysters, clams, and other food safe in summer. They are much better if you give them until autumn (starting with September). In addition, the natural phenomenon known as Red Tide can affect the edibility of certain shellfish (clams and mussels). Red Tide is actually a reddish blanket of billions of microorganisms floating on top of the ocean. The microorganisms, which may appear along the Pacific, Northeast and Florida coasts during the summer months, are poisonous. Any shellfish that eat them become poisonous in turn. In rare cases the toxons produced by Red Tide have even caused death.

    Oysters make you feel sexy. It would seem logical to assume that there is something in seafood, iodine perhaps, which adds to potency, but the truth is that there isn't one particular food that enhances sexual performance. The only thing that really does is an adequate diet, which might as well include oysters.

P

perspiration.

Perspiration "cleans out the pores." Perspiration is the body's response to overheating; it helps cool you down as it evaporates on your skin, but it has no effect whatsoever on internal cleanliness.

See also COLDS, EXERCISE, FEVER.

pickles.

Eating pickles and milk together can make you sick. The idea is that the acid in the pickles will curdle the milk. And who wants to eat curdled milk, right? Actually, the natural secretions in your stomach (stomach acid) will curdle the milk anyway the minute it is swallowed, so eating pickles and milk together doesn't mean a thing, one way or another. If that's your dish, eat, eat.

pimples.

Never squeeze a pimple between your nose and

upper lip. Whenever you squeeze an infected pimple, you run the risk of liberating bacteria into the surrounding tissues. Ordinarily, this can make the infected pimple worse, but it won't really cause much more serious damage. However, the area around the nose and above the upper lip is lined with blood vessels which drain directly into the brain, so squeezing a pimple in this area can, theoretically at least, send bacteria into the blood vessels, and from there into the brain, where they might cause severe and possibly deadly infection. The chances of this actually happening are small, but they are real, so the folk prohibition against fooling around with infections in the middle of your face makes real sense.

plants.

Don't sleep in a room with plants. At night, they will use up the oxygen and asphyxiate you. The myth of the smothering plants is based on the fact that at night when there is no light to trigger photosynthesis (or the production of food), plants *respire.* That means that they begin to break down the food they produced during the day. To do this, they must take in oxygen and then give off carbon dioxide as a by-product. But the amounts of each which they take in and release are so minuscule that you could, if you chose, spend your nights in a greenhouse without worrying about the effects.

So how come the nurses often take plants and cut flowers out of hospital rooms at night? Well, there are two possibilities. The first is that the nurses, who are people like the rest of us, may believe the myth. The second and more sensible reason is that cut flowers sitting in water, which is a perfect breeding ground for germs, are not the best thing to have around sick people. Nor are plants, which can be host to all kinds of crawling things. Even if you are hooked on the real thing, when it comes to a gift for a friend who is sick, maybe the silk or plastic variety is more considerate.

poisoning, antidotes for.

Burnt toast, milk of magnesia, and strong tea are a "universal antidote." The theory behind this widely accepted remedy, which was invented by a toxicologist in the 1930s, is threefold: (1) The charcoal in the toast is supposed to absorb poisons, while (2) the milk of magnesia coats the stomach with a protective layer, preventing absorption of poisons there, and (3) the tannic acid neutralizes alkaline poisons. Unfortunately, the facts are that (1) the charcoal in burnt toast is not at all the same as *activated* charcoal, a specially manufactured agent which does absorb some poisons; (2) milk of magnesia does not prevent the absorption of poisons from the stomach or keep them from burning the esophagus on the way down; and (3) tannic acid may be toxic to a liver damaged by poisons.

Use an alkali (such as baking soda) to neutralize an acid poison (such as a bowl cleaner). No. The combination of the acid and the bicarbonate, or baking soda, can cause the release of carbon dioxide, a gas that can distend the stomach, which has already been injured by the acid, causing it to rupture. The result may be peritonitis.

Use a mild acid (such as lemon juice) to neutralize an alkali poison (such as drain cleaner). Mixing even a mild acid, like vinegar or lemon juice, with the alkali in a drain cleaner can make the temperature of the mixture rise, causing even more damage in the stomach. The sad truth is that there is virtually no antidote for the lye used in most drain cleaners; their action is so harsh that the only certain cure is prevention.

Never induce vomiting if the poison contains a petroleum distillate like kerosene. Standard practice in labeling has been to warn against causing vomiting when a child swallows a product containing petroleum distillates because of the fear that the chemicals would be inhaled into the lungs. However, the newer theory is that it is more important to get the chemical out of the stomach than to worry about inhaling the poison while vomiting it up.

Milk is a safe antidote for most poisons. Wrong. If the poison in question is phenol, camphor, or kerosene, milk can increase its absorption into the bloodstream from the stomach. And, if a child has swallowed a caustic poison such as drain cleaner, the milk may coat the sides of the throat and hide the extent of damage from an examining physician.

With wood-alcohol poisoning, or other poisoning requiring vomiting, give salt water and repeat until the vomit is clear. Salt water may or may not induce vomiting (sometimes it doesn't), but if you give too much of it, you can upset the body's salts/water balance, causing dehydration, salt poisoning, and, in rare cases, death.

poison ivy.

"Leaves of three, let them be." Right. The leaves of the poison-ivy or poison-oak plants may be long or short, shiny or hairy, oval or elongated. They may have smooth edges or saw-tooth ones, and their colors may change with the season (green in spring and summer, pink, yellow, or red in the fall). The plants on which they appear may be low bushes or sturdy vines, and they may flourish in either damp forests or dry and rocky places. But one thing that never changes is the number of leaflets grouped into each leaf. If there are three, don't pick the pretty plant.

The first exposure to poison ivy causes the worst rash. Like all other allergic and allergic-type reactions, the poison-ivy rash is a result of your sensitivity to an allergen in the plant, in this case urushiol, an oily substance which is found in every part of the plant, from the berries to the roots. Your first exposure is likely to be the sensitizing one and therefore mild. In fact, it's the next one that you have to watch out for.

Eating the leaves of the plant makes you immune to poison ivy. This folk remedy, sometimes attributed to the American

Indians, probably has its origins in the fact that somebody once did eat the leaves and never got poison ivy after that. The catch is that the person who ate the leaves probably wasn't allergic to poison ivy in the first place; not everyone is. If a sensitive person eats the leaves (which confer no immunity whatsoever), he would likely suffer a serious allergic reaction, perhaps even requiring hospitalization to deal with it.

Poison ivy is contagious. There is no way to pass poison ivy along from person to person merely by personal contact with the poison-ivy rash. The rash can only be acquired through contact with the exudate of the poison-ivy plant. Of course, if scratching has infected the original allergic rash, the infection can be handed on.

You can catch poison ivy by touching the clothes of someone who has it. While this may sound more far-fetched than the idea of catching the rash by touching it, the truth is that it is not only possible, it happens all the time. The oily substance from the plant which causes the poison-ivy rash can cling to clothes or to anything else which it touches, including the handle of a tennis racquet, bicycle tires, or even the family dog. So, if you put on a sweater which has come in contact with the plant and hasn't been washed since then, it is fairly likely that if you are sensitive to poison ivy, you will end up with a characteristic rash.

You can catch poison ivy from air. Another one with the sound of fiction about it, this is definitely possible. If you burn poison-ivy plants, for example, the allergen in the plant can become airborne, traveling reasonable distances on floating ash or soot. Should you breathe this ash, or find the soot on your skin, you may very well be in for an attack of poison ivy.

Scrubbing with soap and water cures poison ivy. Soap and water are helpful only as a preventative. Use them right away, to wash the poison-ivy allergen off your clothes and skin. Once the rash has appeared, repeated washings can only irritate your already itchy, sore, and irritated skin.

potatoes.

Rubbing a cut potato on face or hands will soften the skin. What you are doing, of course, is applying a light layer of starch, which feels smooth and soft so long as it is moist. Be careful not to leave the starch on too long (never put makeup on over it) or it will dry uncomfortably and may cause itching.

A cut raw potato can soothe itchy skin. It's the starch again, and so long as you aren't allergic to potato starch it may soothe irritated skin. Remember, though, that this is strictly a first-aid treatment, and that the starch should be washed off completely with cool water.

Rinsing the hair in the water from boiled potato peelings will darken it. Some people say that this works because the water is simply dirty from the potato skins, but it is at least theoretically possible that some of the minerals leaching out of the nutritious potato skins may add several layers of darkening particles to the hair. Commercial "hair color restorers" work just this way, depositing layers of a mineral, usually lead acetate, on the hair.

You can remove warts by rubbing them with a cut raw potato. Warts are caused by viruses and do not react one way or another to potatoes. However, since there is some evidence that warts do respond to the host's psychological state, if you really believe that potatoes will cure your warts, why, then, they just might.

Green potatoes are poisonous. A lot of the foods we eat contain minute amounts of substances which, in the pure state—and in much larger amounts—are poisonous. A good example is shrimp, which, like some other foods, contains traces of arsenic, though certainly not enough to do you any harm. The poison peculiar to the potato is solanine, a substance which (in much higher concentrations) gives the deadly nightshade mushroom its punch.
Most of the solanine in the potato plant is in the green part, the

stalk and the leaves, which should never be eaten. There is a tiny bit of solanine in the potato itself, in or near the skin—but so little that it is safe to eat as many potatoes, skin and all, as you wish.

Sometimes the normally brown skin of the potato may have green patches. This does not mean that the potato is unripe, but simply that it has been exposed to too much light. A potato with green patches may taste bitter but if you cut the patches off, it can be eaten safely.

pots and pans.

It is dangerous to eat foods cooked in (stainless steel) (aluminum) or (copper) pots. There are a number of metals that are dangerous if you ingest large amounts of them, and that is why many people believe that cooking in various kinds of pots can be dangerous, too. Whether or not any one pot is a potential source of trouble depends entirely on what it's made of and what you cook in it.

It is not true, for example, that scouring pots made of stainless steel will free particles of nickel, chromium and other metals, which then fall into your food. Nor is it necessarily true that it is dangerous to cook in aluminum pots, although cooking highly acid foods in aluminum will turn the metal dark, which is why you should always cook stews or other dishes containing wine and vinegar (and sometimes tomatoes) in enameled or glass pots.

Unlined copper pans, though, can present a real danger. Copper is necessary to life in minute amounts but toxic if you get too much if it, and a century ago, when unlined copper pots and pans were widely used, copper poisoning was fairly common. Today, all copper pots are tin-lined. They should be relined whenever they show signs of wear so that no copper can leach from the pot into your food; that goes for copper teakettles, too.

Interestingly enough, not all the metals which may leach out of a pot are dangerous. In fact, some people speculate that the changeover from iron to other kinds of pots and pans may be one of the reasons for the rising rate of iron-deficiency anemia among American women. Aside from the fact that women simply ate more in the days when iron pots were used, and thus got more iron from the diet (it is practically impossible for a woman of childbearing age to get enough iron from a 1,500-2,000-calorie diet), iron from the pot itself would leach into the food. Eaten, it could help to raise the body's iron level and thus help to prevent anemia. Today we substitute iron pills for the iron pots. Somehow, it lacks romance.

pregnancy.

A missed period is a sure sign of pregnancy. Not necessarily. The menstrual cycle can be interrupted by a lot of things, including emotional upset, physical trauma, or illness. It usually takes at least two missed periods to prove that conception has taken place, and even then it's a good idea to have a backup test done (a gynecologist can usually tell simply by physical examination at that point) to be certain that the interruption in the menstrual cycle isn't due to some other cause.

Strange food cravings are normal during pregnancy. They are certainly common, but whether or not they are normal is a matter of some dispute.

The obvious physical explanation for these cravings is that they represent the body's need to satisfy some nutritional deficiency. The desire of poor Southern mothers to eat clay during pregnancy, for example, has been laid to an iron deficiency; a craving for ice cream or milk may represent a calcium deficiency. A lot of psychologists, however, don't buy that view and some feminists are on their side. In fact, feminist writer Simone de Beauvoir said more than twenty years ago, in *The Second Sex,* that pregnant women showed hysteria and childish obsessions in their food cravings. Others have said that women use their food cravings to cut down on their husbands' freedom during their pregnancy or simply to show their resentment of the pregnancy itself. The idea is that since the woman is inconvenienced by the burden she is carrying, the man should go through some inconvenience too, even if it is only the legendary trip through a midnight snowstorm in search of, say, pickles and mango-banana ice cream.

While such things sound funny at first blush, they may be serious for the pregnant woman and her baby. Too much ice cream, for example, can cause her to gain too much weight; too many pickles and other salty delights may contribute to the development of toxemia, which is dangerous for both the mother and the child; and, as for clay or laundry starch, too much of these can cause anemia or block the intestines.

Pregnant women are "eating for two." Yes and no, depending upon exactly how you translate "eating for two." If you mean that a pregnant woman has to consider her developing child when she chooses the foods she eats, then the answer is an unequivocal yes. A well-balanced diet is a virtual necessity if the mother wants to produce a healthy baby; pregnancy is not the time to stick to a soft-drink-and-candy regime. On the other hand, if you take "eating for two" to mean doubling the calories, then the answer is an equally unequivocal no. An adult woman who is not pregnant should be eating about 2,000 calories a day to maintain her normal weight. A pregnant woman can push that up to about 2,400 calories a day, and (according to figures from the National Foundation/March of Dimes) she will gain about 22 to 27 pounds. She should then produce a baby which weighs in at about 7½ pounds (obviously, this varies), which is a good weight at which to begin facing the world.

You never really go back to your pre-pregnancy weight once you've had a baby. Not true, although it is an admittedly spiffy excuse for getting comfortably fat as you get older. If you have gained between 22 and 27 pounds in pregnancy, you should lose about 18 to 20 pounds in the first week after the baby is born and the rest of the added weight within a month after delivery. (Just for the record, this is exactly what having the baby added to your weight: 7½ pounds for the child, 6½ pounds for the fluid surrounding the child in the uterus and about 6 to 10 pounds in fat and water scattered throughout your body.)

Women lose a tooth for every child. There is some evidence that hormonal changes during pregnancy can alter the chemistry of the mouth, making it more acid. The increasing acidity may make cavities more common, but proper dental care and scrupulous cleansing every day can go a long way toward helping the pregnant woman avoid decay, not to mention tooth loss.

During pregnancy, the growing fetus takes calcium out of its mother's teeth. Fetuses need calcium to build their own bones and teeth, and, if the mother's diet does not contain ample amounts of such calcium-rich foods as milk and cheese, along with the Vitamin D to speed their absorption into her body, the fetus may begin to absorb calcium from the mother's skeleton. Experts disagree, however, on whether or not the fetus will ever absorb calcium from its mother's teeth, and, in any event, the entire situation can be easily avoided with proper diet.

It's not safe to have intercourse during pregnancy. Although there are, naturally, many exceptions, in most cases it is safe to have sexual intercourse during virtually every stage of pregnancy. One general exception seems to be the last two weeks to two months of the pregnancy, when, some doctors believe, both the act of intercourse and of female orgasm may increase slightly the possibility of a premature birth.

Pregnant women are rarely sexually aroused. On the contrary, research by sex therapists Masters and Johnson has shown that pregnant women experience a higher rate of sexual arousal. The reason, according to Masters and Johnson, is simple: there is extra blood in the pelvic region during pregnancy and the engorgement of blood vessels is a sensation normally associated with sexual excitement.

See also CIGARETTES, CLAY, VD.

prenatal influences.

A pregnant woman's cravings and/or fears can show up as physical marks on her baby. For example, a strawberry birthmark on the child shows that the mother loves strawberries (or hates them); a woman frightened by a cat can give birth to a child with a cat-shaped birthmark. No. Period.

A pregnant woman can influence the intellectual development of her child by engaging in cultural experiences during pregnancy. If you take this to mean that a woman who loathes classical music can produce a musical child simply by listening to symphonies through nine months of pregnancy, forget it. On the other hand, a woman who truly enjoys music will have it in the house after the child is born, and, growing up in a musical environment, the baby is more likely to have positive attitudes toward it. The point is simple: children pick up (or discard) their parents' sincere preferences and dislikes in real life, after birth, not in the womb.

Wearing high-heeled shoes while you are pregnant can cause the baby to be born cross-eyed. No way, although wearing very high heels while pregnant can cause the mother to end up with a backache from trying to balance the forward-thrusting weight of her body on the heels.

Eating "cold" foods, like ice cream or sherbet, can cause the baby to catch cold in the mother's womb. In some Latin countries, "cold" foods also include citrus fruits and some vegetables. Neither these or really cold desserts, however, have any influence on the baby, who, like any other human being, would have to come in contact with a cold virus to catch a cold.

Never eat citrus fruits while pregnant. They are acid and will burn the baby. Too many oranges, lemons, and grapefruit, like too much of other food, may disagree with your stomach, but in moderation these fruits can do you and your baby nothing but good since they supply Vitamin C and various other necessary nutrients. In addition, lots of fresh fruits and vegetables can help alleviate the common constipation of pregnancy.

If you exercise or raise your hands above your head, the baby will strangle on the umbilical cord. There is no way at all that any movement of your body during pregnancy can influence the positions of the child and umbilical cord. Of course, if you are going to lift your hands over your head to put something on a shelf, it is better not to do it while perched precariously on an unsteady chair, because there is always the possibility that you will fall and break a leg. Even if you do, however, your baby has a good chance of continuing undisturbed, so securely is it cushioned within the uterus.

If you sleep a lot, the baby will end up stuck to your back. Not a chance, not even if you sleep flat on your back all the time.

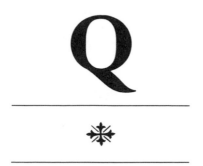

quicklime.

Burying a body in quicklime will "destroy the evidence." Although it has long been regarded as the perfect murderer's helper, at least in mystery novels, quicklime (also known as lime or calcium oxide) only does the job halfway. A strong alkali, it will dissolve soft tissues such as skin and flesh, but it won't do a thing to hard tissues or bone. Cover a body with quicklime, and you will end up with a perfectly preserved skeleton, similar to those of prehistoric animals or people caught naturally in lime when they tumbled into a sticky pit or were covered with lava from an overflowing volcano.

quince.

Boiled quince seeds heal burned or irritated skin. When simmered or boiled, the seeds of the quince yield fatty oils and gums which make a nice, mucilaginous dressing. There is no solid evidence at all to indicate that this dressing is of any medical value in treating burns, although it may make healthy (but dry) skin slightly softer. The gum can be used medically as a stabilizer or suspending agent, and is often used the same way in cosmetics. People who like to make their cosmetics from "natural" sources sometimes use the gum from simmered quince seeds as a hair conditioner, before setting.

R

rainwater.

Wash your hair in rainwater for an "extra-clean" feeling. Water from wells is "hard" or alkaline; it contains minerals, notably calcium and magnesium, which can leave a film on your hair. Water from surface reservoirs is "softer," or more acid, but because it is, it can corrode the pipes through which it travels to your tap, carrying minerals with it along to your hair.

Rainwater, on the other hand, is relatively "pure." It is non-alkaline and nearer to the pH, or acid-alkaline balance of your hair. You have to use *country* rainwater, though, since rain falling in the city will pick up soot and other goop from the air through which it falls. And you've got to use the rainwater as you collect it. Leaving it to collect and sit in a barrel only guarantees that there will probably be a scum of bacterial growth on top when you go to use it.

redheads.

Redheads have terrible tempers. Some do, some don't,

but almost all tend to exhibit rather freely the blush or redness of face which we have come to associate with rage. It works this way: When you are angry or excited, the minute blood vessels under the surface of the skin tend to fill with blood. If you are a brunette, or sometimes a dark blond, this will show as a faint flushing. If you are a redhead, however, your skin will usually be so thin that the blood in the surface vessels shows through. What looks like a minor blush in others will look like "purple" or "red" rage in you, and, if it happens often enough, people accustomed to associating that flush with anger will conclude that you do have a terrible temper.

regularity.

It's normal to move one's bowels once a day. In this, as in everything else, individuals differ. Several movements a day may be normal for one person, while another normally experiences only one movement a week; most of us are obviously somewhere in between. There is no such thing as an absolutely "normal" pattern, though, except what is normal for you.

The older you get, the less regular your bowel movements will be. Constipation is a common companion of old age, but increasing one's consumption of bulk foods (vegetables, fruits, and grains) can help things considerably.

Irregularity causes poisonous wastes to pile up inside your body. Unless the irregularity is caused by a malignant growth or blockage of the intestines, it poses no immediate danger or possibility of internal poisoning. However, there is increasing speculation that infrequent elimination may allow food to degrade or oxidize within the body so as to liberate potentially carcinogenic substances. For this reason, diets high in bulk or laxative foods have gained new popularity, as possible preventives against cancers of the digestive tract, specifically the colon and rectum. In addition, there has been some theorizing that anti-oxidants, such as Vitamin C, may also help prevent intestinal cancers by keeping foods from combining with oxygen within the digestive tract. Absolute proof of both theories remains in the future.

See also LEMON JUICE

rosemary.

Rosemary causes miscarriages. This herb is an *emmenagogue,* which means a medication that can strengthen uterine contractions and help expel menstrual discharge. Obviously small amounts used in food won't work therapeutically. It would require a medically prepared distillation, or enormous amounts of the herb itself. Actually rosemary's reputation as an abortifacient is probably a fake, since it is more likely that the herb has helped to "bring on" the menstrual periods of women who weren't really pregnant to begin with.

rubella.

see GERMAN MEASLES.

S

✲

---

salt.

Don't pour salt on open wounds. A good idea. The salt creates an osmotic effect, pulling water out of tissues around the wound so that they shrink and pull. This can be very painful indeed. (It's not generally known that sugar does exactly the same thing.)

seeds.

If you eat fruit seeds, a tree will grow in your stomach. This myth has all the earmarks of something picked up from a child's book of fairy tales. The bottom line, of course, is that if you eat seeds in almost every case they will be quickly and smoothly excreted from the body. However, there are some seeds that can be dangerous, which means that they are poisonous, not that they will implant in the stomach. The kernels of peach and apricot seeds, for example, contain cyanide, and they can, if eaten in sufficient quantity, be fatal. In fact, there have been fatalities reported in children who ate sixteen or seventeen dried apricot kernels sold as health food. (It is the kernel of the apricot which is used to make Laetrile, the alleged anti-cancer drug whose active principle is cyanide, which is supposed to destroy the cancer cells without harming the healthy ones.)

sex determination.

The position in which you have intercourse or the day of the month on which you indulge can determine the sex of the child. Superstitions about time and position actually have a grain of truth in them, for they all draw, however inadvertently, on the differences in motility between male and female sperm cells. Directly put, the male cells are better swimmers. They can make their way faster through thick vaginal mucus. Therefore, if you want to conceive a boy, you should have intercourse on days of the menstrual cycle when the vaginal secretions appear thick and sticky. If you want to conceive a girl, however, you should have intercourse on days when the vaginal secretions are thin and slippery, since this increases the chance that female sperm cells will make their way safely to the uterus.

As for position, you can get a good argument going here, since it seems perfectly clear that any position that delivers sperm cells right up against the cervix will either (1) make it even easier for the fast-swimming male cells to reach the ovum, or (2) increase the chances that the slower-moving female cells will get there first. It's important to note, of course, that neither of these methods is anywhere near foolproof. Far from it.

However, you can raise the odds by employing artificial insemination. In studies done at New York University Medical School in 1960, doctors were able to predict the sex of the unborn child with up to 80 percent accuracy when the woman conceived via artificial insemination. Couples who used the timing methods at home were able to produce boys at will only about 68 percent of the time; for girls, the successful-prediction rate was about 10 percent lower.

Tying off the right testicle (or the left) before or during intercourse will produce boys (or girls). This superstition goes all the way back to Hippocrates, who, like a lot of other people, believed that boys were produced by one testicle and girls by the other. Actually, Hippocrates was ahead of his time in attributing the determination of a child's sex to its father, since most early theorists tended to blame the mother for girls and praise the father for boys— which explains why wives who did not bear sons were often dispensed with. However, while the sex of the child does depend on the male (he supplies both male and female sperm cells), both kinds of cells are produced in both testicles. Interfering with one or the other will have no effect at all on a man's ability to father either boys or girls, always provided he can function at all under such trying circumstances.

Carrying a baby high (or low) shows whether it is a boy (or a girl). There is no relationship at all between the child's sex and the position it occupies as a fetus in its mother's womb. Occasionally, however, a doctor can predict the sex of an unborn child from its heartbeat, since the heart of an unborn girl child consistently beats just a little bit faster (about five or six beats a minute) than that of an unborn boy child. The method, needless to say, is not foolproof. The only absolutely certain method of predicting a child's sex prior to its birth is amniocentesis, a procedure by which some of the cells in the amniotic fluid surrounding the fetus are withdrawn from the mother's womb. The test is used to determine the presence of severe birth defects and genetic malfunctions such as Down's Syndrome (mental retardation) and Tay-Sachs disease, among others. The cells that are withdrawn from the amniotic fluid for this test also show the child's chromosomal makeup and offer positive proof of gender.

sex organs.

The size of a man's (nose) (hands) (feet) indicates the size of his penis. Scientifically speaking, there is no statistical correlation whatsoever, nor is there any relationship between the size of a woman's mouth and her sexual organs.

A large penis is more sexually satisfying for a woman than a small one. The vagina is an elastic organ which can stretch to accommodate a large penis or tighten to enclose a smaller one, so that there is no physical reason at all for size to have any impact on sexual satisfaction.

Black men have larger sex organs than white men. Although the genitals of black men may appear larger when flaccid than those of Caucasians, when erect, all penises fall within the same general range (average: about 6¼ inches in length when erect), which varies by individual, not by race.

sexual intercourse.

Sex is dangerous for people who have had heart attacks. Because the heartbeat accelerates during intercourse (up to about 130 beats per minute from the normal rate of 60 to 80 beats per minute), many people fear that sex is too much of an exertion for them if they have suffered heart attacks. However, no scientific study has ever shown a notable correlation between sexual activity and heart attacks, and researchers at the Downstate Medical Center in Brooklyn, New York, have even shown that the increased heartbeat during intercourse can be controlled through regular exercise. That is, regular exercise can keep the heart rate steady, even through the exertion of intercourse.

Regular sex cures acne. There is no indication that this is so, but there may well be a correlation between the age at which most people start to experience sex on a regular schedule and the age at which adolescent acne starts to fade. Both are likely to happen around the early twenties, and, once upon a time, some observant person almost certainly put these two facts together as an easily believable cause and effect.

Frequent sexual intercourse cures infertility. On the contrary, it may even impede a man's ability to father a child (although it won't interfere with his ability to have sex). It takes about forty hours for the sperm count to return to normal levels after each act of intercourse. Therefore, frequently repeated intercourse is actually a kind of natural contraceptive technique—though it has

enough failures to warrant its being approached with extreme caution, and probably not at all by people who really don't want to
conceive.

sexual potency.

   *Masturbation or too frequent intercourse can make a
man impotent.* No, although both can make him temporarily less
fertile.

   Repeated sexual intercourse "saps a man's strength."
This myth is based on the erroneous belief that a man's "strength"
resides in his seminal fluid and that the supply of this fluid is finite.
Neither, of course, is true.

   *Athletes should avoid sex (a month) (a week) (the day)
before a match or game.* Stripped of its magic aura, sexual
intercourse is really nothing more than an athletic exercise and, while
common sense dictates against sex fifteen minutes before a match or
game (common sense also dictates against playing four sets of tennis
right before competition), there is no scientific reason at all to avoid
sex while training.

   *There is an age after which men are invariably
impotent.* No, but men who think that this is true may find that, for
them at least, it is. On the other hand, men who are willing, and who
have willing partners, will usually be capable of erection and intercourse as long as they live, even up into their eighties and nineties.
The trick is not to allow oneself to get out of practice, since neglected
sexual powers are hard to coax back to life.

   "Prostate trouble" always makes men impotent. It is
true that prostate surgery was once considered a virtual death
sentence insofar as sexual potency was concerned. But newer surgical
techniques allow a man to attain erection even after prostate surgery.
In some cases, however, the seminal fluid will not be ejaculated at
orgasm, but will instead go back into the bladder. This will make no

real difference either to the man involved or to his partner, although it's certainly going to be unsettling at first.

shellfish.

Shellfish are bad for your skin. Perhaps. Shellfish are high in androgens, as are organ meats (such as liver) and wheat germ. Androgens are sex-related hormones which can cause the oil glands to produce more than their normal complement of oils, leading to blocked pores and, ultimately, acne-like eruptions. All of us produce androgens, and taking in more from our food may be just the trigger required to set off a round of skin problems.

Shellfish and liquor are a deadly combination. They can be, but only if you are allergic to shellfish to begin with. The alcohol lowers your resistance to allergens, and even if you could take, say, a few forkfuls of lobster without showing a reaction, combining those forkfuls with a drink or two might just be too much for your immune system. In all fairness to shellfish, however, it should be noted that taking alcohol with anything to which you are allergic will increase your chances of experiencing an allergic reaction.

shingles.

If shingles go all around the body, you will die. Shingles, or herpes zoster, is a virus disease characterized by blisters which usually show up in a line halfway around the upper trunk. Ordinarily, the shingles will occur on only one side of the body, but, in rare cases, the line of blisters will complete the circle. As anyone who has ever had herpes knows, it can be quite painful, and when the shingles go completely around the body, the pain may be doubled. But herpes in and of itself has never been known to be fatal, although, since it tends to develop when the body's defenses are lowered by emotional trauma or serious illness, it may turn up in connection with an ultimately fatal illness.

showers, cold.

A cold shower can kill sexual excitement. True. It's a matter of the body's trying to concentrate on two major sets of stimuli at once. The cold shower will win out every time.

A cold shower is stimulating first thing in the morning. Actually, shocking might be a better way to describe it, and, in some cases, the shock can be positively dangerous. Dr. Roderick W. Childers of the University of Chicago points out that a really cold shower decreases the pulse rate and increases the blood pressure. If you put this increased strain on your heart after you have been overheated—by exercising, say, or when you get up out of a warm bed—the doctor, a cardiologist, says that it is equivalent to revving a car up to about forty miles an hour and then abruptly shifting into reverse. In other words, a real cruncher, which, in rare instances, might even trigger a heart attack.

A cold shower will sober you up in a hurry. Like the stimulation of the caffeine in a cup of coffee (or the more modern equivalent, a whiff of oxygen), a cold shower may wake you up, but it won't eliminate the alcohol from your blood system, and, until time does that, all you will be is a "wide-awake drunk." It is simpler (and kinder) to let people sleep the whole thing off.

silence.

"Silence is golden." There is literally no end to the list of the possible malignant effects of excessive, continuous noise. (A sudden loud boom may make you jump, and, if it is loud enough, may deafen you temporarily, but the real culprit is the noise which goes on and on.) Studies on both human and animal subjects have shown that noise can make your blood vessels constrict, make your muscles tense, disrupt your kidney functions, force hormones into your bloodstream, and, not surprisingly, cause deafness by making the inner membranes

of the ear swell. One animal study even suggested that loud, continuous noise could cause impotence and sterility. The question is, how much is too much? Well, for comparison's sake, the lowest sound the human ear can hear without aid is probably measured as one decibel. A lover's whisper, heard from a distance of about five feet, registers around 30 decibels; normal conversation hits 70; a symphony orchestra in full flower can hit 130; and a modern jet bottoms out at about 160.

sinuses.

People get sinus attacks when the weather is (cold and damp) (cold and dry) (warm and wet) (hot and dry) (changeable). Yes. Anatomically speaking, a sinus is simply a hollow space or cavity in a bone. What most people mean when they complain about sinus trouble, though, is the sinuses in the skull, right around the nose and eyes. Each of these cavities is lined with mucous membrane, which, like the mucous membranes in the nose, mouth, and throat, secretes a constant flow of sticky mucus. Ordinarily, this secretion drains out of the sinus cavity through a narrow passage to the nasal cavity. If that passage is blocked, however, the mucus will build up in the sinus, the mucous membrane will become irritated and a vacuum may create painful pressure within the sinus itself. There are any number of things that can cause the sinus passages to swell and close. Among them are extremes of weather, changes in weather and barometric pressure, and, of course, allergies. The truth is that there is virtually no climate on earth which is guaranteed to help you avoid sinus problems.

Air conditioning causes sinus problems. If you turn the air conditioner on too high, yes, it can cause an allergic reaction which will make the mucous membranes in your sinuses and sinus passages swell. However, air conditioners, used intelligently, can also help cut down on sinus problems by filtering out allergens from the air in the room.

Steam heat causes sinus pain. If the steam heat makes the room too dry, that can, in turn, dry up the mucus in your sinus passages and cause blockage of the drainage system. If you use steam heat, use a humidifier too, to keep the humidity in your home at a comfortable level.

Smoking causes sinus trouble. Tobacco smoke can paralyze the tiny hairs, or cilia, in your nose. When that happens, they stop beating back and forth. Since the main function of the cilia's movement is to filter dirt and germs out of the air you breathe in through your nose, anything that slows them down can allow that stuff in. And once it's inside your head it can irritate the mucous membranes in your sinuses, and there you go again.

Swimming in a pool can cause sinus attacks. If the water in the pool is chlorinated, it can irritate the mucous membranes inside nose and sinuses, tripping off the whole sinus syndrome.

skin color.

Two white parents with a hidden "black" gene in their background can suddenly produce a blackskinned child. Skin color is the result of more than one gene. Almost all of us have some lighter and some darker skin color genes in our makeup and our skin color reflects this mixture. It is possible for two relatively lightskinned people to pass on their darker skin color genes to a child and to produce a baby which is relatively darker than they are. But it is not at all possible for very lightskinned people to produce a very darkskinned baby (or vice versa). The real clue to this long-lived myth lies in the definition of black and white skin colors. In societies such as the ante-bellum American South or modern South Africa where even the hint of color is considered a social catastrophe, the slightly darker child is labeled "black"—but only in the eyes of the color-conscious. In the real world, such minor differences are so unapparent as to be irrelevant.

Pale skin is a sign of anemia. Sometimes yes; sometimes no. Most frequently, pale people simply have thicker skin, which hides the surface blood vessels that give color (including the "blush") to the thinner-skinned people. A much more reliable indication of anemia is the presence of such clearly clinical symptoms as lowered hemoglobin, or the absence of color from the inside of the mouth, the eyelids, under the nails, or the creases of the palm.

See also FINGERNAILS.

sleep.

Most people need eight hours sleep a night. On the average, yes, most of us do require about eight hours sleep in order to be awake and alert the next day. To be specific, about 60 percent of us need the magic eight hours. The rest of the population get along on anything from two hours a night to twelve hours, with just as many people going along at one end of the spectrum as at the other. Sleep differences, of course, are strictly individual. They vary among members of the same family and rarely cause any problems except perhaps when someone who can get by on five hours sleep sets up housekeeping with someone who needs ten.

"Early to bed, early to rise, makes a man healthy, wealthy and wise." Maybe in the good old days, when most people worked farms, getting to bed early made sense since it let you get up early with the animals. Today, however, there is more leeway for personal style in earning a living and, anyway, there is no health benefit at all in going to bed early. What counts is that you get the sleep you need. *When* you get it is irrelevant.

One hour's sleep before midnight is worth two after. Other than the fact that daytime sleep may sometimes be interrupted by noises which are absent at night, the time of day you get your sleep has nothing whatsoever to do with the quality of the sleep, so long as you establish a particular sleeping pattern and stick to it. According to some research done at Johns Hopkins University, this may be of crucial importance for adolescents. The levels of growth and thyroid-stimulating hormones rise when you go to sleep; so do the levels of sexual hormones in adolescent girls. The researchers at both Johns Hopkins and the Sleep-Wake Disorders Unit at Montefiore Hospital in New York theorize that adolescents who do not follow regular sleep patterns may not grow normally or may experience delayed puberty, and that the small size and delayed puberty of abused children may well be due to their parents' keeping them from sleeping regular hours. Even adults, who no longer are actively growing, may be disturbed and disoriented if normal sleep patterns are interrupted.

"I slept like a log." Some people move around more than others, but everybody moves at least a bit during even the best night's sleep, and nobody at all ever got through an entire night's rest just lying there, "like a log."

"I didn't sleep a wink all night." The truly sleepless night is a remarkable exception, brought on by illness or worry or a combination of the two. Chronic insomniacs, the ones who complain that they never sleep at all, almost always turn out to be people with perception problems, not sleep problems. They may feel as though they never get to sleep, but time after time, when observed under scientific conditions, in laboratories or in their own homes, they fall asleep, usually within a half hour of getting into bed. No scientific study ever performed has been able to validate any insomniac's claim that she has been existing for years without sleeping.

Counting sheep puts you to sleep. Believe it or not, there is now a study, conducted by two psychologists at Harvard University, which proves that watching those sheep leap over fences in your imagination really may be an effective way of tricking your active brain into letting you fall asleep at night. Why? Because visualizing the sheep engages the energies of the right side of your brain, thus preventing it from creating other more disturbing thoughts. Counting, on the other hand, is a function of the left side of the brain, and prevents it from coming up with other problems that require rational, concentrated thought and might well keep you wide awake solving them. In other words, counting sheep as they dance through and over fences keeps both sides of your brain too busy to disturb you and the result is—you fall asleep.

sleepwalking.

Waking a sleepwalker can drive him mad. Waking a sleepwalker can cause confusion and disorientation as he tries to figure out where he is and how he got there, but it will not cause madness or even serious confusion. Nevertheless, if possible, it makes more sense to guide the sleeper right back to bed, from which he is less likely to arise a second time. Undisturbed, he will probably go right back to deep sleep; awakened, he may be up the whole night trying to figure out what happened.

smile.

A smile uses fewer muscles than a frown. Right. And you thought it was all propaganda for one of those smile-button manufacturers.

snakebite.

Whiskey is an antidote for snakebite. Both alcohol and snake venom lower blood pressure, so feeding whiskey to a snakebite victim can only increase her chances of going into shock. The only real antidote for snakebite is an antivenin, a substance which contains antibodies to counter the effects of the venom. Most antivenins, however, are prepared from horse serum, to which a significant number of people are allergic. Late in 1976, three researchers at the University of Utah and the Veterans Administration Hospital in Salt Lake City, speculating on the fact that herpetologists have known for at least a century that the blood of certain snakes, such as the rattlesnake, contain antivenin factors, began to work with rattlesnake blood as a potential source of an antidote for a rattlesnake bite. This antidote would not have the allergic problems associated with antivenins prepared from horse serum. It would be useful not only in the United States (where there are only about 1,000 rattlesnake bites and 30 resulting deaths each year), but in areas of India and Africa where there are many times that amount.

If a snakebite victim moves fast or gets excited, the venom will spread faster. It is true that anything that speeds circulation or starts blood pumping to the muscles (as excitement or excited movements do) can help the snake venom spread more quickly. But the real reason for staying calm is so that you can take the intelligent action, which means, whenever possible, getting to a doctor or hospital where you can get the appropriate antivenin.

Cross-cut the snakebite wound and suck out the venom. It's always a good idea to get the venom out of the wound so that it cannot circulate through your body. However, a deep "cross-cut" (which is two small slashes that criss-cross each other across the wound) may do more harm than good, adding another injury to the original one. A much better idea, according to the experts at a "Snakebite Symposium" held in 1978 at Louisiana State University, is to make two small shallow parallel cuts on the site of the puncture. Then suck out as much venom as you can (you'll usually get 50% or more). Even though snake venom isn't a stomach poison, don't swallow it; spit it out and wash your mouth out, too. Apply a loose tourniquet-type band to the bite wound—loose enough to allow a finger to slip under it—and, once again, get to a hospital or doctor as quickly as possible.

sneakers.

Sneakers are bad for your feet. Once upon a time, when the word "sneakers" conjured up an image of canvas-topped shoes with rubber bottoms and no steel shank, there was a large germ of truth in this saying. Those old-fashioned sneakers didn't give the foot any support, and the plain rubber bottoms didn't allow for much evaporation for sweat. Today, however, there are sneakers with steel shanks and some with suede or even leather uppers. If you didn't see the sign saying "Sneakers," why, you might think they were comfortable "shoes," no worse for your feet than any other kind of shoes and certainly a lot better than vinyl ones, which allow no evaporation of perspiration at all and can make your feet smelly and uncomfortably hot to boot.

See also ATHLETE'S FOOT.

soap.

Soap is gentler on the skin than detergents. It depends on the soap. And on the detergent. Obviously a laundry detergent, loaded with bleaches and whiteners, is too strong for personal use. (Indeed, it is sometimes too strong for laundry use; some people react with itching and rashes if they wear clothes or sleep on sheets washed in detergents.)

However, detergent preparations made for personal use can often be gentler on skin and hair than pure soap products, which are, after all, made from fatty acids and alkalis. The new "baby shampoos," for example, don't make a baby cry because they are made of detergents which don't sting the way soap does if you get it in your eye. Most bath "soaps" are actually detergents; check the label on yours. If there is a long line of chemicals (some of them ending in the letters "—ium"), that's the detergent. Plain soap bars don't have to list their simple ingredients because the FDA assumes that everyone knows, or is supposed to, that soap means fatty acids and alkalis. (Extras, like antibacterial ingredients, do have to be listed on the label, and so does perfume.)

You can catch germs from soap bars in public places. Damp soap bars which never quite dry out are pleasant places for bacteria to grow in; you can pick up the bugs when you pick up the soap. That, along with the economy of a measured amount, is why most public restrooms and gyms use glass or metal dispensers at the sink.

sore throat.

Wrapping flannel soaked in turpentine around your throat cures a sore throat or cold. The warmth of the flannel can make you feel a little more cozy and relaxed, but it won't do a thing to shorten the length of your cold. Neither will the turpentine, although it can take your mind off a sore throat and stuffy nose. Since the solvent is a counter-irritant, it will irritate your skin slightly, making it feel warmer, and the turpentine fumes will irritate the lining of your mouth and nose, seeming (for a short time) to clear a path through the mucus. Both skin and mucous membrane effects, however, are short-lived. You'd do better to inhale the warm steam from a vaporizer, which won't cause the skin irritations some people suffer from turpentine dressings.

spanish fly.

"Spanish fly" makes you feel sexy. "Spanish fly," which is more properly known as cantharides, is a kind of beetle which, when ground up and applied to the skin or taken by mouth, can produce an itching, burning sensation, and in males, this irritation may actually produce an erection. (For women, it's just uncomfortable.) Of course, there are drawbacks to this kind of self-deception. Cantharides is extremely toxic when swallowed or absorbed through the skin. If the dose is large enough, it can cause severe gastric upset, kidney problems, collapse, and, occasionally, death, all of which are a high price to pay in search of a little pleasure.

spinach.

Spinach makes you strong. There *is* iron in spinach, but, despite all those Popeye cartoons you saw as a kid, there isn't all that much. In truth, there are only about 3 parts of iron to every 100,000 parts of spinach, and your body can only absorb about one-eighth of that.

That means that, in order to get all the iron she needs from spinach alone, an average adult woman would have to eat as much as twice her weight in spinach every year. And any woman who had the fortitude to do that would find herself with problems she hadn't bargained for. Spinach contains oxalic acid, which is what gives it that bitter taste, and too much oxalic acid can concentrate in the urine, producing kidney stones.

Finally, would you believe that all those kids who turned their noses up at cooked spinach really had a scientific point? This is the story. Spinach, like a number of other foods, contains nitrates, the same chemicals which are used to preserve things like ham and frankfurters. Under normal conditions—that is, as long as the spinach is raw—the nitrates in there are presumably harmless. But, when you cook spinach, you have to be extremely careful to serve it immediately and to serve it piping hot, because if you allow it to sit around and to cool off to the lukewarm temperatures, the nitrates in your spinach may degenerate into nitrites. And nitrites, in combination with various other substances, can turn into nitrosamines, the potential carcinogens that have turned so many people off meats like ham and hot dogs.

sprains.

Put a (hot) (cold) compress on a sprain to make it better. Yes. The trick is to use the right one at the right time. First comes the cold compress, to keep the tissues around your sprained ankle or wrist from swelling and to reduce the immediate pain. You can keep using cold compresses for a day or two, then switch to the hot compresses, which also relieve pain. If you were to use the hot compresses first, you would risk the chance of making the tissues swell more, because heat increases the flow of liquids (both blood and water) into the tissues.

spring.

"In the spring a young man's fancy lightly turns to

thoughts of love." According to one study, conducted in Paris by chronobiologist Alain Reinberg, the level of male hormone production is highest in the fall, and, with more testosterone, or male hormone, surging around the body, the level of male sexual activity naturally rises.

If that doesn't square with your experience, it is only fair to note that chronobiologists—persons who study body rhythms—sometimes disagree, and many believe that there is also a peak of hormonal activity in the spring.

spring tonic.

Like your house, your body needs a "spring cleaning." Years ago, when fresh fruits and vegetables were not readily available through the winter, people may well have been starved for the natural roughage which keeps the digestive system running at top speed. When spring came, with its promise of new crops, it may well have seemed logical to purge the body of the "poisons" accumulated through the winter months. In point of fact, it wasn't necessary at all, and violent purging may even have been harmful.

Sulfur and molasses cure "spring fever." If the lassitude and dreaminess of "spring fever" were really anemia in disguise, sulfur and molasses might have at least a small effect. Molasses is rich in iron, not to mention chromium (a trace metal essential to the metabolism of carbohydrates), and calcium. It also contains some sulfur (which is necessary for the metabolism of proteins). Of course, mixing sulfur with molasses gave the stuff a bitter taste, which let everyone know it was a medicine. And since sulfur has laxative effects (it's used today as a veterinary laxative), it helped to purge the body.

stuttering.

Forcing a naturally left-handed child to use his right hand will make him stutter. There is no real proof either for or against this supposition, but it is at least theoretically possible, since it seems logical to assume that stuttering may be the verbal equivalent of reaching for something with the left hand and then stopping in mid-air to switch to the right.

However, if this were true, then we might expect to have a lot more stutterers than we actually do. Modern studies almost always show that at least 90 percent of the people in the world are right-handed and a careful examination of historical art and artifacts appears to show that this has always been so. (One draws such conclusions by counting how many people in paintings are shown using the left or right hand, by examining implements and weapons to see which hand they were made to fit, by scrutinizing skeletons of men killed in battle to see how many were injured on the left side, indicating attacks by right-handed warriors, and so forth.)

Yet the possibility exists that the right-handedness is an acquired rather than an inherited trait. In experiments performed at Jackson Laboratory in Bar Harbor, Maine, for example, mice placed in bias-free situations (feeding tubes could be reached with either the right or the left paw) divide into equal numbers insofar as the use of one or the other paw is concerned. When behaviorist Robert L. Collins altered the situation so that the mice *had* to use either the left paw or the right one, about 90 percent of the mice conformed to the bias, whichever it was.

Since that is about the percentage of people who conform to our right-handedly biased society it seems possible, not to say likely, that more of us begin as lefties than end up that way. Obviously not all of these formerly left-handed people stutter, which means that something more than forced right-handedness is at fault.

Stutterers outgrow the problem. Sometimes yes; sometimes no. There is no hard and fast rule.

Tickling a baby's toes can make the child stutter. It's hard to talk when you are laughing, so a laughing baby may appear to stutter, but the effect is strictly temporary, disappearing as soon as the tickling ends.

sugar.

Sugar causes cavities. It contributes to the decay process. Sugar is acid and provides food for the bacteria in the mouth which cause tooth decay and periodontal disease. In addition, the acid sugar itself may help to eat away at your teeth.

Sugar (or candy) makes your cavities ache. What aches isn't the cavity; it's the dental tissue around it. When you push sugar into the hole in your tooth (the cavity), it sets up an osmotic reaction, pulling fluids from the surrounding tissues into the sugar concentrate, creating pressure which makes the tooth ache. It's pretty much the same thing that happens when you put salt on an open wound.

See SALT.

Sugar is "empty calories." Unlike most other carbohydrates, such as fruit or grains, sugar provides no nutrients except calories—there are no vitamins, no minerals, no fats, no proteins. Since virtually all other foods provide these nutrients along with their calories, or energy units, they are always a better food bargain than sugar. (NOTE: The "empty calorie" charge applies only to sugar on its own. When sugar is mixed into a food which contains other ingredients, that food—even if it is candy—does contain some basic nutrients, although it is true that you may be able to get more nutrients for less calories from foods made without sugar.)

Sugar is quick energy food. All carbohydrates contain sugars of one kind or another, and every time you eat a carbohydrate food, such as fruit or grain, the sugar travels through your bloodstream to the liver, where it is converted into glycogen. When you need energy in a hurry, your body will call upon reserves of this liver glycogen, which is then sent out into the muscles. If you eat an adequate diet, you will always have adequate glycogen reserves for the ordinary exercise you are likely to run into, up to and including a fast game of tennis. (Marathon runners, and other professional athletes, however, may have to supplement their glycogen reserves for their extraordinary efforts.) The sugar you eat right before a tennis game or an exercise session is quickly metabolized and moved right into available storage in your body.

Eating too much sugar causes diabetes. Because diabetics have to cut down on their intake of sugar, many people assume that sugar is the cause of their condition in the first place. Actually, although diabetes has been around since the earliest recorded times, nobody really knows exactly what causes it, although it is assumed to be genetically influenced. The only role which sugar might play in its cause is to make people fat. Fat people have a harder time than skinny ones in using insulin to burn up their bodies' stored glucose, and this may contribute to the onset of diabetes in overweight people who are genetically predisposed to the disease.

Eating too much sugar causes heart disease. A matter of speculation with absolutely no scientific proof that it is either true or false.

Brown sugar is more healthful than white. Raw sugar, which is the first product of the crushing of sugar cane, contains syrup (molasses) and sugar crystals, which are ultimately refined into ordinary table sugar. This first product contains the nutrients of molasses: some minerals and vitamins, including iron. But raw sugar is banned in the United States for the simple reason that it is unsanitary, since it can contain insect bits and droppings, as well as industrial contaminants, molds, and bacteria.

The final product we get from processing raw sugar is table sugar, stripped of all nutrients. In an attempt to get a better product, nutritionally speaking, many people opt for brown or "turbinado" sugar. Turbinado sugar is partially refined raw sugar; brown sugar is ordinary white sugar which has been sprayed with molasses syrup. Although both look more nutritious, brown instead of white, the extra nutrients are virtually undetectable because the nutrients in the sugar plant simply aren't present in the parts used to make refined sugar and commercial molasses.

The sugar in fruit is more healthful and natural than table sugar. Plain white table sugar or sucrose comes from a plant and is just as authentically "natural" as the fructose in fruit or the lactose in milk. What makes the difference is that the sugars in foods come coupled with the other nutrients in the foods, while table sugar comes alone and has to be added to foods (which already have their own sugars) in order to gain any real nutritional value.

suicide.

People who threaten suicide never really go through with it. Believing that is rather like believing that barking dogs never bite, and anyone who has been bitten by a barking dog can tell you how foolish that is. Actually, people who plan suicides are very serious about it, even to the point of trying more than once. For example, statistics reported by Dr. Earl Grollman, editor of *Concerning Death: a Practical Guide for the Living* (Beacon Press), show that fully 12 percent of those who try suicide and fail try again within two years and succeed.

Despite figures like that, most people persist in the notion that suicide warnings are fake and even that people who die as suicides really didn't mean to. Considering the fact that there is a reported suicide every twenty-six minutes in the United States, the denial of the reality of suicides and suicide warnings says more about most people's inability to cope with suicide than it does about the reality of suicides and suicide warnings, every one of which should be taken with the utmost seriousness.

Most suicides occur in the dead of winter. The true suicide season appears to be spring, when all those bursting buds and burbling birds are just too much for people who barely made it through winter. Every major study of suicide trends has shown this to be true; in one study undertaken by a German scientist, the suicide rate peaked later in the year as one moved north from Greece. The correlation with a later spring seemed obvious.

(As if that were not enough, statistics processed by computer in a University of Minnesota study showed that the incidence of depression and of ulcer attacks also rose with spring. April, alas, may really be the cruelest month.)

sunburn.

Getting a bad sunburn is one fast way to get a tan. Tanning is the result of the dispersion of melanin, a color agent, throughout the skin. Some people do not have enough melanin in their skins to tan at all, and some people have enough melanin to look dark at all times, from olive right through the darkest of "black" skins.

Sunburn, on the other hand, is an injury caused by exposure to the ultraviolet rays of the sun. The skin's reaction to a severe sunburn is exactly what it would be to any other kind of burn. First, the heat of the sun causes the surface blood vessels to dilate, increasing the flow of blood through them. This increased flow of blood makes the walls of the blood vessels more likely to leak. At the same time, the irritation of the ultraviolet rays can cause the breakage of small enzyme packets in the skin. When these packets break, the enzymes spill out, causing swelling of the skin and the collection of fluid. (The reaction is similar to what happens inside the nose and throat of an allergic person who is exposed, say, to ragweed or pollen.) If the burning is severe enough, the skin will blister. The entire syndrome can cause injuries lasting from two days to two weeks, depending upon the severity of the burn. Far from giving you a base on which to build a tan, this kind of injury makes the skin more vulnerable to the sun, and requires that you take extra care once the worst symptoms have disappeared.

Any oil will protect you from the sun. On the contrary, sunburn preventives (sunscreens or sunblocks) are one class of cosmetics which cannot be duplicated cheaply at home. "Baby oil," which is commonly plain mineral oil, offers no protection at all against the sun's burning rays; most vegetable oils will do for you what they do for a chicken—that is, set you up to be broiled. Just about the only home remedy that offers any protection at all is sesame-seed oil, which, it should be pointed out, is only about a third as effective as any commercial product.

See also IODINE.

sunglasses.

Wearing sunglasses indoors can weaken your eyes. Wearing very dark sunglasses all the time can, possibly, make you more sensitive to light, so that you would be uncomfortable for a time if you stopped wearing the shades. However, your eyes will readjust as soon as you give up the dark glasses, and there are situations in which lightly tinted glasses are extremely useful indoors. For example, if you work all day in an office with fluorescent lighting, you will be more comfortable and even see better wearing glasses with a very light tint to them. Fluorescent lighting operates in the blue-green part of the spectrum, a harsh, discomforting light by which to read and work. In addition, fluorescent lighting is not a steady source of illumination. It flashes on and off as many as sixty times a second. While this "flutter" is too fast to be perceived consciously by the human eye, the subliminal effect is one of irritation and discomfort. Tinted glasses can make the blue-green light more bearable and can, at the same time, soften the irritation of the fluorescent flutter.

swimming.

Wait an hour after eating before going into the water. So long as the meal in question isn't a seven-course banquet, heavy enough to make you sleepy, there's no reason at all not to swim right after eating. In fact, swimming after you've eaten makes a lot more sense, physiologically speaking, than swimming before eating. When you are hungry, your muscles are hungry also, starved for the glycogen, or fuel, which your body manufactures from the food you eat, and, as any serious athlete knows, glycogen-starved muscles are much more likely to cramp. The admonition to "wait an hour" after eating is an instinctive bow to the fact that there will be more glycogen available to you then, but your system will have quite enough to get you going long before the hour is up. Enjoy it.

swimming pools.

You can become pregnant by swimming in a coed swimming pool. Only if you do in the pool what most people do in more comfortable surroundings.

The water in swimming pools turns blond hair green. If the blond is artificial, it is possible that a chemical reaction between the chlorine in the pool water and the bleached hair will produce a faint greenish tint. It is also possible, though, to watch your hair turn a bright green even if you never go near the (pool) water. In a series of cases reported in the *New England Journal of Medicine* and *Science Digest* late in 1975, the culprit turned out to be ordinary fluoridated tap water. The fluoride in the water system in Framingham, Massachusetts, acidified the town's water, and as the acidified water passed through copper pipes, it picked up traces of the metal, which, in turn, produced an "epidemic" of green hair at Framingham State College. The green turned up in everyone's hair, brightest in the blonds'.

See also ATHLETE'S FOOT.

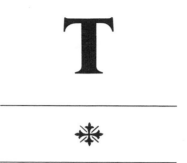

T

tea.

    Tea has less caffeine than coffee. That is almost certainly true, although some types of tea have more than a respectable amount of caffeine, and the longer you brew them, the more caffeine you get in the cup. If you change the statement to read, "Tea has less *stimulants* than coffee," though, the answer would be, false. In addition to caffeine, tea leaves contain theine, an alkaloid that stimulates the body exactly the same way caffeine does. Too much tea can keep you awake at night exactly the way too much coffee does.

    Tea soothes your stomach. This is obviously an outgrowth of the belief that tea contains less caffeine than coffee. Once you know that tea contains theine, and that it contains a lot of tannic acid and tannin, both of which can irritate your stomach, you can easily understand why ulcer patients and some people with other stomach disorders are warned off tea as well as coffee. (In fact, simply drinking a lot of tea, say, up to eight or nine cups a day, can cause you to experience symptoms which remarkedly duplicate the stabbing, burning pains of an ulcer.)

Wet tea bags or compresses of cool tea can soothe burned, irritated, or itchy skin. Yes. Here the tannic acid or tannin which can cause turmoil in your tummy calms and heals the burning or itching sensation. So long as you are not allergic to the tea itself, this may well be a nifty home remedy for sunburn or other minor skin problem.

teeth.

Healthy teeth are white. The normal color of teeth is faintly yellowish, or, to put it more kindly, ivory. No one has absolutely white teeth (although the darker your skin, the lighter your teeth will look by comparison), and the very best dentures recognize this fact—if you scrutinize them closely, you will see that they too are ivory, not white. Nevertheless, most people still believe that their teeth should be white, and a lot of toothpastes and powders use that as a selling claim, promising to make your teeth "whiter than white." Dentifrices which really do affect the color of your teeth are either abrasive enough to remove deep stains, in which case they are abrasive enough to scratch your teeth, or they contain a kind of white "paint" which covers up stains.

Some people have soft teeth. This is often used to explain why some people have more cavities than others. However, since dental enamel is the second-hardest substance on earth (only diamonds are harder), the real reason is far more likely to be either bad dentistry or rotten home care. The one exception: people whose individual body chemistry is such that bacteria grow more freely in their mouths, making the oral cavity acid and literally eating away at the teeth. Even then, however, the cause is not the softness of the teeth, but the strength of the attacking agents.

See also AGING, PREGNANCY.

temperature.

Normal body temperature is 98.6° F. Actually, that's more like an average than an absolute, since the normal temperature of the human body varies considerably with age, sex, and even the time of day. Infants and young children, for example, run an average normal temperature which is around 99° F. or even slightly higher (and may spike a fever as high as 104° F. during a seemingly minor illness—and show no ill effects from it). Older people, on the other hand, run an average normal temperature around 97° F. In the course of a month, a woman's normal temperature varies with her menstrual cycle and will rise about a degree right after ovulation. Finally, most people begin the day with a temperature lower than that with which they go to sleep. (People who wake up each morning and hop out of bed as though they were going to a fire often are—their own. Their body temperature rises more quickly in the morning than does that of slugabeds.)

No matter what time of day it is or what day of the month, if you take your temperature by sticking the thermometer under your arm, you will find that it runs about a degree or two lower than if you take your temperature by mouth, and about two degrees lower than if you take it by rectum.

See also HANDS, COLD.

tetanus.

You need a tetanus booster every two years. That used to be the medical routine, but more recent research has shown that the immunity conferred by the tetanus shot may last for as long as ten years. Some experts even theorize that, after the childhood series of tetanus-diphtheria-pertussis shots, immunity may last as long as thirty years.

Every puncture wound requires a tetanus booster. It depends on the seriousness of the wound and the time elapsed since your last shot. If you had a shot a year ago, and the puncture wound was made by a relatively "clean" instrument (like a kitchen knife or a carpet tack), many doctors believe that no new shot is needed. On the other hand, the tetanus organism is a spore which is found in open fields contaminated with animal wastes, so if you step on a nail out there, your doctor is likely to give you a booster just to be sure.

Stepping on a rusty nail causes tetanus. A rusty nail is dirty, but it isn't, in and of itself, a cause of tetanus. The real problem lies with the conditions under which the nail (or any other piece of metal) rusted. Usually, rusty objects are found out of doors, in gardens or fields, where the tetanus spores abound. It is the transfer of the spores that causes tetanus; if you step on a rusty nail indoors, you can get a nastily infected wound, but the chances are you won't get tetanus.

thunderstorms.

Thunderstorms turn milk sour. It is certainly possible (some people would say, virtually certain) that milk left standing around during a thunderstorm will turn sour. But that has nothing to do with the noise of the thunder or with random electricity zapping through the air. Rather it has to do with the fact that micro-organisms such as bacteria multiply like rabbits in the hot and humid weather which comes with thunderstorms. These micro-organisms turn milk sour if they are allowed to grow unchecked in the liquid. Depending on the bacteria involved, the soured milk can be nutritious and delicious (yogurt, for example) or it can be "spoiled" and dangerous.

Thunderstorms make you feel edgy or sexy. Normally, the earth's atmosphere is negatively charged, but, as a thunderstorm approaches, it builds up a positive charge on the ground below and for several miles around. The attraction between the positive charge under the storm cloud and the normal negative charge in the cloud can make the air between "crackle." In addition, as the barometric pressure drops and the storm approaches, the human body responds by absorbing moisture. This produces a pressured, edgy feeling somewhat akin to that which some women feel in the days before their menstrual periods begin, when the tissues of their body are similarly soggy. Between the electricity in the air and the water in the body, it is certainly possible to feel edgy and slightly jittery, a condition that might sometimes be confused with sexual arousal.

Don't use the telephone during a thunderstorm. Because their wires are good conductors of electricity, telephones and a number of plug-in appliances (like hair dryers and electric razors) can turn into electrical hazards if outside wires are hit by lightning. Obviously there is less danger of this happening in a city where the wires are underground, but the National Weather Service warns that even in those cases the possibility exists that your electrical appliances may turn savage during a thunderstorm.

Thunderstorms make your hair stand on end. Yes, the interaction between the positive charge in the air and the negative charge in the thunderstorm cloud *can* make your hair stand straight up (it works best, of course, on crewcuts). When that happens, or when your skin suddenly feels tingly, drop to the ground and make yourself as flat as possible, because the tingle means that lightning may be about to strike you.

toenails.

Always cut toenails straight across. If you do that, you will leave sharp corners on the nails which can catch in your socks or stockings or, when you put your shoes on, nip into the skin folds at the side of the nail. A much better bet is to cut the nail in a slightly rounded curve and then smooth down the edge so that there are no rough snares. Remember, though, that moderation is important: don't make a deep cut at the sides or file into the skin.

tonsils.

Tonsils are useless and should be removed. Tonsils may indeed be useless. There has been some indication that they may be part of the bodily defense system which protects us against infection, but this has never been conclusively proven. What is known, however, is that modern antibiotics can often deal quite nicely with infected tonsils. Since there is no such thing as a truly minor operation—the use of general anesthetic *always* involves the possibility of death—it usually makes sense to attempt to treat tonsils medically first, rather than rushing in with a scalpel to remove them. Of course, tonsils should always be removed if they make it hard for a child to breathe, if they are continually infected, or if they appear to be malignant.

Removing the tonsils prevents sore throats. If the sore throat is caused by infected tonsils, taking them out (when necessary) will certainly cure the sore throat. However, a team of researchers at the University of Pittsburgh School of Medicine has come up with evidence to show that tonsillectomies are rarely justified simply because a child has a bad year of sore throats. The researchers followed 65 youngsters who had a history of frequent sore throats (7 in one year, 5 in each of two consecutive years, or at least 3 in each of three consecutive years). What they found was that less than one-fifth of the children (17 percent) were likely to have as many sore throats again. That is, a child who had as many as 6 or 7 sore throats in one year was unlikely to have as many the next, even with his tonsils still in place. The obvious conclusion: frequent sore throats are no reason to take out a child's tonsils (always provided that the sore throats don't involve abscessed tonsils).

trench mouth.

"Trench mouth" is catching. Not only isn't it catching, it isn't even "trench mouth." The disease—bleeding gums, loose teeth, bad breath—got its name during the First World War when soldiers

in the trenches in France began to exhibit all the nasty symptoms. Since there were so many of them, packed in so close together, it was assumed that they were catching trench mouth from each other. In time, however, dentists learned that trench mouth is really a variety of periodontal disease which is brought on by poor hygiene and conditions of stress. Given sleep, proper food, and toothbrush and floss, any simple case of trench mouth can be more or less easily dispensed with. (If there are infections in the mouth, some antibiotics will often be required.)

tuberculosis.

A skin test which is positive for TB means that you have the disease. Not necessarily. Most of us are exposed to TB bacilli at some point in our lives and may harbor the germs on our skin or in our bodies for years without ever developing the disease. The positive skin test simply indicates the presence of the bacilli and is so unreliable as an indicator of illness that the FDA announced in 1977 that it was going to ban the test entirely. Much more reliable is the sputum test, which shows the presence of the bacilli in the lungs, or a chest X-ray, which can reveal the presence of "hidden" or "quiet" lesions on the lungs.

tuna fish.

Tuna fish causes acne. Tuna fish is one, but by no means the only, food which is rich in iodides—and iodides can cause pustular reactions, or eruptions on the skin. Some of the other foods rich in iodides are: artichokes, cabbage, seaweeds, other saltwater fish, sea salt, and spinach.

Never eat tuna fish salads away from home. Actually, there's no reason not to eat tuna fish salad at your Aunt Kate's house, but there is some danger in eating a tuna fish salad just any old place. The culprit is tuna fish plus mayonnaise. Unless the mayonnaise mixture is refrigerated properly, it can be a perfect breeding ground for bacteria and a very common source of mild food poisoning, which is why these salads should never be added to the picnic basket.

turista.

You only get turista in tropical places. Not true. The miseries of *turista*—vomiting, diarrhea, fever—are caused by an organism called *E. coli,* which lives in all food and water, not to mention the human digestive tract. You get the disease, which is sometimes called Montezuma's Revenge, when you run into a group of strange *E. coli,* different from those you usually live with. If, for example, you live in New York, you can get a mild case of *turista* from the water in any other large American city, and vice versa. The difference is that in that case you'd probably attribute your symptoms to nerves or to something you ate rather than connecting it with water, a connection which would be made automatically if you were traveling in, say, Mexico or the Caribbean.

Drinking bottled water will protect you against turista. Only if the water was boiled before it was bottled. If your bottled water is simply bottled local water which hasn't been boiled, it isn't going to do anything good for your tummy. Nor will carbonated beverages or local beers, unless the water used in them has also been treated. (On the other hand, carbonated beverages, even locally bottled ones, will help protect you against cholera because carbonation tends to slow the growth of cholera organisms.)

Always peel fresh fruit before eating it to avoid turista. If the fruit is contaminated with *turista*-causing organisms, simply peeling it won't do any good at all. The minute you cut the skin, you've spread any organisms on the surface to the inside fruit itself. Much safer to stick to cooked fruits and vegetables. But they have to be thoroughly cooked; just dipping them in prettily simmering water won't do. For the best protection, boil your vegetables vigorously, like your water for tea or coffee, for about fifteen minutes.

See also YOGURT.

twins.

Twins run in families. Identical twins do not; their birth is always a result of the accidental separation of one fertilized ovum into two distinct individuals. (Incomplete or partial separation produces Siamese twins, which do not run in families either.) Fraternal twins, on the other hand, do tend to run in families. The reason is obvious: the birth of fraternal twins results from the fertilization of two separate ova. Since most women only release one egg at a time, the tendency to release two eggs is extraordinary and assumed to result from an anomaly in the reproductive system which is, more likely than not, inherited. (There is some speculation that the trait may be passed on to a woman from either her mother *or* her father's side of the family.)

Identical twins are identical. To all intents and purposes, they are biologically alike. Their blood types are the same, as are their eye coloring, skin coloring, and fingerprints. Skin grafts between them will take without any problem of rejection at all. In addition, identical twins have been shown to share levels of intelligence and to develop the same diseases at roughly the same time in life, even when they were brought up completely separate, one from the other.

In a set of fraternal twins with one male and one female, the female is almost always barren. This appears to be true among cows, where the female half of a set of fraternal twins (she is called a free martin) has only about a 5 percent chance of conceiving. But it is absolutely not true for human beings.

Older women are more likely to have twins. This is not true in the case of identical twins. The chances of having fraternal twins, however, do rise as a woman gets older. Women who are twenty years old, for example, produce fraternal twins at the rate of about 4 pairs of twins in every 1,000 births. By the age of forty, a woman's chances of having twins rises to about 16 pairs of twins in every 1,000 births, and, after 40, the rate begins to decline.

A woman's chances of producing fraternal twins also increases with the number of pregnancies she experiences; the chances of producing twins after four pregnancies, for example, is much greater than the chance of producing them the first time out.

Fat women are more likely than thin ones to bear twins. This appears to be true insofar as fraternal twins are concerned. The reason for the higher rate of twin births among heavier women appears to be that they (the heavier women) have a higher level of sex hormones in their bodies and are more likely to release two eggs at one time.

Twins are slower intellectually than singly-born children. It has long been observed that, in early childhood, twins learn to talk later and have lower IQs than children born one at a time. Now researchers at the University of Calgary in Canada have come forth with an explanation for the phenomenon. Using television recorders to tape the home lives of forty-six sets of twins and single children, all about two and a half years old, the researchers found that the reason lay not with the twins but with their mothers. Mothers of singly-born children have more time to spend with their babies and are likely to stimulate them to talk earlier in life. Mothers of twins, on the other hand, have literally to divide their time in half, and, in addition, because they assume that the babies will amuse and stimulate each other, they often tend to leave the children on their own for longer periods of time. The conclusion, according to psychologist Hugh Lytton, was that simply spending more time with the twins would improve both their IQs and the rate at which they began to speak.

U

※

ulcers.

People with ulcers should drink plenty of milk and cream. The rationale behind this time-honored remedy was the supposition that milk (or cream) would neutralize the acidity of the stomach, which, it was assumed, had led to the ulcer in the first place. A recent study at the Veterans Administration Hospital in Los Angeles, however, showed that milk (either whole, low-fat, or skimmed) had a minimal effect on the existing environment of the stomach. In addition, it actually stimulated the production of more stomach acid. Finally, milk and cream in quantities can be fattening and may supply more cholesterol than anybody should have.

Ulcer patients should stick to a bland diet. Not necessarily. More and more, modern gastroenterologists are finding that how often the patient eats is more important than what is eaten. Small meals of practically anything you like (within reason, of course—if you couldn't eat raw onions before you developed an ulcer, you can't eat them afterward, either) work just as well as a bland diet was supposed to, and some doctors even say that three normal meals a day work just as well as either.

Ulcer patients need antacids daily (sometimes hourly). While antacids do neutralize the stomach environment, they may have undesirable side effects if used on a daily basis. (See also BAKING SODA.) In addition, there is little evidence that aluminum and magnesium hydroxide, which are the most important ingredients in most over-the-counter antacids, have any effect at all in the healing process when you have an ulcer. Modern treatment is more likely to involve the use of cimetadine, or Tagamet, a drug which cuts down on the secretion of stomach acid. Tagamet has been used in Europe for several years with reportedly excellent effects. It has only recently been introduced into the United States.

People with ulcers should never drink coffee or tea. You can add cola drinks to that list. The offending ingredient is caffeine, which triggers the production of stomach acid. It does this so efficiently that people who don't have ulcers may experience all the symptoms—stabbing pain when hungry and the like—just by drinking too much coffee or tea.

Women don't get ulcers. Now they do. In the last twenty years, the incidence of male ulcers has dropped significantly, while the incidence of female ulcers has risen. Since no one has ever really proven that ulcers come from stress on the job or in the home (many apparent candidates for ulcers never develop them), nobody has yet tried to prove that Women's Liberation is responsible for this increase, but, according to Dr. Morton I. Grossman of UCLA's Center for Ulcer Research and Education, equal rights may be at least partly responsible, since women are now drinking more, smoking more, and generally participating more often in activities which were once reserved for men.

urine.

Urine is an antiseptic. In primitive societies, body wastes are often credited with magical properties and used in healing poultices or medical preparations. Since none of us are so far from the primitive as to forget our superstitions entirely, this is obviously one reason that many of us still believe in urine's antiseptic properties. Another, better reason is the scientific one: urine does indeed have antiseptic powers, since it contains both salt and ammonia. Naturally we are talking about clean, fresh urine from healthy individuals. Urine which has been allowed to stand around has almost certainly been contaminated by bacteria; urine from sick people may already be contaminated. (Urea, a major component of urine, is used commercially today as a preservative and healing agent in many cosmetics and/or medications.)

Gargling with urine heals a sore throat. Well, it is salty and it does have antiseptic properties, but, all things considered, you are probably better off with warm salt water.

Drops of urine in the eyes prevent cataracts. There is absolutely no truth to this myth. In addition, if the urine is contaminated with bacteria, the danger of eye infections is a virtual certainty.

Injections of urine break down the body's fat cells. Absolutely untrue.

V

vaseline.

Vaseline makes hair grow on your face. This heavy hardened oil may mat down facial hairs so that they appear more prominent, but it has no effect whatsoever on their growth rate or pattern. As a skin softener, Vaseline, which is a trade name for petrolatum or petroleum jelly, is a mixed blessing. It is an extremely effective barrier which prevents the evaporation of moisture from the skin, but it is very greasy and it isn't water soluble, so it is hard to remove.

Vaseline is an effective sexual lubricant. It is unquestionably lubricating, but terribly hard to wash off, since it won't dissolve in water. More important, if you use petroleum jelly with a condom or diaphragm, the lubricant will eat right through the contraceptive device, making it worthless.

VD.

Gonorrhea is "no worse than a bad cold." With the

discovery that penicillin cured gonorrhea, it did seem for a while that this form of VD, if detected early enough, could be no more of an ordeal than an ordinary cold. In the past few years, however, more and more cases of penicillin-resistant gonorrhea have been showing up. These cases require more and stronger doses of antibiotics and, while some VD researchers report that a gonorrhea vaccine may be available within a few years, others are grimly awaiting the appearance of a strain of gonorrhea that will prove resistant to antibiotics other than penicillin.

You can catch VD from a toilet seat. It's rare, but it can happen, if the organisms remain alive in the moist discharges which may be left on the toilet seat. Should these discharges come in contact with mucous membranes (vagina, anus, mouth, nose, eyes), the disease can be transmitted to a new host. Once the toilet seat is dry, the organisms will die. They live only in moist, warm environments.

Contraceptives protect you against VD. Some do. Chemicals like foams and creams make the vagina inhospitable for the venereal-disease organisms. The Pill, however, does just the opposite, affecting the lining of the vagina in such a way that it is more friendly for venereal-disease bugs. Plain mechanical devices like the diaphragm, the coil, and the cervical cap don't offer any protection against venereal disease, but the condom does since it keeps the sexual organs from direct contact.

Syphilis and gonorrhea are hereditary. An hereditary disease is one that is passed from parent to child through the genes. Since neither syphilis nor gonorrhea is handed on this way, neither one is hereditary. That doesn't mean, though, that an infected mother can't infect her fetus or newborn infant. If she has syphilis, the bacteria in her bloodstream may pass through the umbilical cord to the child, whom it will attack just as savagely as it attacks an adult human being. More often than not, the fetus of a syphilitic mother will be stillborn. Gonorrhea, on the other hand, is transmitted to the baby during birth, as the infant passes through the vagina. Catching gonorrhea this way was once the single most important cause of infant blindness. Today, newborns are given silver nitrate or penicillin eyedrops to prevent the development of gonococcal conjunctivitis and blindness.

Pregnant women can't get venereal disease. This folk myth is based upon the belief that during pregnancy the cervix, or mouth of the uterus, closes tight to keep the baby from falling out. The supposed shutting of the cervix is also thought to prevent venereal-disease organisms from getting into the uterus and infecting the pregnant woman. In reality, of course, the cervix does not "shut tight"; the baby is attached to the wall of the uterus and, barring trauma, will not "fall out," and venereal-disease organisms do not have to "get into the uterus" in order to wreak havoc. Infection can occur whenever the organisms meet mucous membranes (mouth, eyes, vagina, and anus), and pregnant women are as vulnerable as anyone else.

vinegar.

Vinegar compresses cure a (migraine) headache. A cool, wet dressing often feels good when you have a headache and may even have some (slight) effect in shrinking swollen, throbbing blood vessels near the skin surface. In addition, vinegar fumes are irritating and may divert the headache sufferer's attention from the pain, breaking the tension-pain cycle which characterizes many common headaches.

Drinking vinegar cleans out the body. Like wine, vinegar is acid and can be irritating to the bladder, so that, having drunk some, you will feel the urge to urinate much more frequently. Some people regard this increased urination as a sign that the body is cleansing itself; most people regard it simply as the bother it usually is.

Vinegar rinses make your hair shine. Washing your hair with soap, which is alkaline, can leave the tiny scales, or imbrecations, on each hair ruffled and open so that your hair doesn't reflect light evenly and looks dull. Vinegar, which is acid, can remove any alkaline residue left by soap and also close those tiny scales down tight on the hair, so that any light which hits your hair reflects back off a smooth—that is, "shiny"—surface. However, since virtually every shampoo sold today is made of synthetic detergent and neither leaves an alkaline residue nor ruffles the scales on the hair, vinegar rinses (which may darken blond hair) aren't really necessary.

See LEMON JUICE.

Vinegar and water make a safe cleansing douche. The main virtue of a vinegar-and-water douche is that it is acid enough to maintain the acid environment of the vagina. This ensures the proliferation of "good" bacteria which reside in the vagina and the control of yeast organisms. (When the bacteria population is decimated, usually after a woman has taken antibiotics, the yeasts multiply, causing many of the familiar vaginal infections.) In addition, vinegar-and-water douches don't contain coloring, perfumes, or other chemical additives, which may be either allergenic or irritating. However, no douche can be used effectively as a contraceptive, and frequent douching, even with so simple a mixture as vinegar and water, can dry out the vaginal tissues. In point of fact, the healthy vagina cleans itself. Any substantial discharge is a sign that something is wrong and requires a doctor's attention.

See LEMON JUICE.

virgins.

Virgins can't get pregnant. It is rare, but it is possible that a girl who is technically a virgin (which is to say that she has never had sexual intercourse involving the insertion of the penis into the vagina) may become pregnant.

If a male ejaculates near the vaginal entrance, contact may be so intimate that, even without insertion of the penis, the sperm can gain entrance to the vagina and from there travel to the uterus, where fertilization can occur. Obviously this is not the sort of thing that happens every day of the week, but it can happen often enough to shake anyone's complacency.

The second possibility for virgin pregnancy is more theoretical. Among some animals, females have been known to produce young without the contribution of the male. This phenomenon, called parthenogenesis, occurs when an ovum begins to divide and multiply on its own. In laboratory frogs, an electrical impulse has been used to trigger parthenogenesis. Mammals, however, have never been shown to produce young parthenogenetically, although, in 1974, researchers at the Jackson Laboratory in Maine did show that laboratory mice often produced parthenogenic cells which went on to become tumors or cancers. In 1977, however, these researchers reported that when parthenogenic embryos from two or three female mice were combined and then transplanted into a host "mother," the embryos went on to develop into living animals.

To date, no single instance of human parthenogenesis has been confirmed. If such a thing ever is discovered, the child will be female, an exact genetic duplicate of her mother, since there will have been no contribution from a male parent.

If a woman is a virgin, there will be vaginal bleeding after the first intercourse. Unfortunately for the purists among us, the answer to this one is an unqualified "maybe." It is commonly assumed that a virgin has an intact hymen or membrane covering the opening to her vagina. When this membrane is torn as the penis enters the vagina, there is some bleeding. However, the fact that there is no bleeding at all does not necessarily mean that the woman was not a virgin. Hymens can be stretched in any number of ways, including the insertion of a menstrual tampon, so as to permit easy entry of the penis. In addition, even a normal, intact hymen may not necessarily cover the vaginal opening completely. Obviously, there has to be at least a small opening so that menstrual blood can escape. Less obvious, though, is the fact that hymens, like every other feature of the human body, differ and even a virgin may have a hymen with an opening large enough to allow the penis to enter without tearing it and thus without causing any bleeding.

Virgins never have orgasms during their first intercourse. They may or they may not. It is all a matter of individual reactions. Whether or not a woman experiences orgasm is no proof one way or the other as to whether or not she was a virgin.

vitamins.

Natural vitamins are more healthful than synthetic ones. It is always better to get your vitamins in their truly natural state—that is, in food. That way, you get a logical combination of nutrients, another way of saying "a balanced diet." If your idea of vitamins, though, is a vitamin pill, then there is no difference whatsoever between the "natural" and the "synthetic" ones, at least insofar as your body is concerned. Chemically, the two are identical. You may, of course, find differences from brand to brand, a different filler here, a different form of the vitamin (pill, tablet, liquid) there. But the major difference between natural and synthetic vitamins is the price tag.

Vitamins are natural substances which are safe no matter how much of them you take. Stuff and nonsense. Repeated large doses of Vitamin A can produce symptoms similar to those of brain tumors. Overdoses of Vitamin D can interfere with the workings of your kidneys. Large amounts of Vitamin C can be transmitted from a pregnant woman to her fetus so that the fetus is born requiring larger-than-normal doses of Vitamin C simply to keep it from developing scurvy. In extraordinarily large amounts (anywhere from three to ten times the FDA's recommended daily allowances), vitamins have to be regarded as medication rather than simple dietary supplements, and should be treated with the respect you would accord any other medicine.

vitamin A.

Vitamin A prevents cancer. For years, nutrition writer Adelle Davis, who died of cancer in 1975, had insisted that massive doses of Vitamin A were able to stop the growth of cancerous tumors in laboratory rats, sometimes even causing them to disappear. Ms. Davis recommended massive doses of the vitamin daily for human beings, but the drawback is that in large amounts Vitamin A can produce serious side effects.

It may have seemed surprising, therefore, to read recently that the National Cancer Institute in Washington, D.C., has now requested permission from the FDA to test certain forms of Vitamin A on persons who are at high risk of cancer of the bladder, breast, and uterus, to see if the vitamin really does have the preventive effect it has seemed to have in laboratory animals.

However, the Vitamin A which the National Cancer Institute proposes to test is a *synthetic* form of the vitamin, called 13-cisretinoic acid which, unlike "natural" Vitamin A is not fat soluble and thus cannot be stored in the body, building up so to cause the side effects normally associated with overdoses of the vitamin in the form in which it is sold in your local drugstore. Whether or not the synthetic form of the vitamin will work to prevent cancer must wait upon the formal experiment, but the possibility is certainly intriguing.

And it certainly will give the lie to the idea that the only valuable vitamin is a "natural" one.

vitamin B$_{12}$.

Vitamin B$_{12}$ shots give you fast energy. If you have a Vitamin B$_{12}$ deficiency (which would show up as hardening of the arteries or a loss of hair color, though not the normal graying which accompanies aging), then a shot of Vitamin B$_{12}$ would certainly be in order. Otherwise, it is really of no value to you.

Deficiencies of the other B vitamins can produce such things as berberi (Vitamin B$_1$, or thiamine), dimming of vision (Vitamin B$_2$, or riboflavin), pellagra (niacin), nausea and morning sickness (Vitamin

B₄, or pyridoxine), premature aging (pantothenic acid), fatigue (folic acid), and muscular disorders (Vitamin B₁₅, or pangamic acid). In all these cases, however, the symptoms can be reversed by correcting the diet, since there are so many foods rich in the B vitamins. Among them: eggs, flour, beef, milk, chicken, molasses, and yeast. In the most dramatic example of the reversal of vitamin-deficiency disease in this country, for instance, public-health officers were able to wipe out pellagra in the American South simply by including whole grain wheat in the victims' daily diet. No additional supplementation was necessary.

vitamin C.

Vitamin C prevents colds. No formal, scientifically arranged experiment has ever shown that large doses of Vitamin C are able to cut down on an individual's tendency to catch colds, although in some experiments, conducted with employees of the National Institutes of Health in Bethesda, Maryland, it did appear that the vitamin was able to relieve the symptoms very slightly or to shorten very slightly the duration of the cold once it was caught.

vitamin E.

Vitamin E prevents heart disease. Numerous researchers over the years have run numerous studies to see whether claims that Vitamin E prevents heart attacks can be substantiated. One of the most recent studies involved 48 angina pectoris patients in Baltimore who were each given 1,600 I.U. of Vitamin E a day to see if the vitamin would improve heart function. The researchers could find absolutely no evidence that Vitamin E had helped the hearts to function better or had relieved the symptoms of the disease, which is precisely what virtually every other scientifically devised study of Vitamin E and heart disease has shown, as well.

W

warts.

Warts can be cured by (spells) (radish juice) (the juice of marigold flowers) (raw meat) (copper pennies) (burying a potato) (the sap from dandelion flowers) (a black snail) (bacon) (the bark of an ash tree) (saliva) (burying a bag with as many stones as you have warts) (etc.) Yes, no, and maybe. Like many skin conditions, warts seem to respond to a change in the patient's psychological state. A patient who believes in the power of spells, voodoo, magic, or the juice of marigold flowers may very well find that his warts can be cured by any one of these or a dozen other specifics. In one strictly scientific test a few years ago, physicians at Massachusetts General Hospital in Boston hypnotized seventeen patients once a week for five weeks, telling them that their warts would disappear. After three months, six of the group lost all their warts, and three more got rid of up to 75 percent. In a control group, with no treatment at all, not one patient lost even one wart.

See also FROGS.

water.

Drink eight glasses of water a day. Taking in lots of liquids (nonstimulating drinks such as fruit juices will do as well as plain water) really does help to keep your system in tone. For example, the fluids will serve as a digestive aid, bulking up wastes so that they are eliminated more quickly. That's why eight glasses of water a day are usually regarded as a way to avoid constipation. Second, the copious fluids will keep your kidneys flushed and help you empty your bladder often. Since most bladder infections result from urine remaining too long in the bladder, where bacteria can multiply, the fluids both prevent infection and help alleviate those which occur anyway. Finally, water can be used as a diet aid, since it is noncaloric but "filling" enough to fool your stomach into thinking it has been fed. (Warm water is more filling than cold; add a dash of lemon juice to make it more palatable.)

Chlorine purifies drinking water. Not completely. Chlorine kills large numbers of bacteria in water, reducing them to levels which are ordinarily harmless. However, if you use an aerator or a water filter on your faucet, and neglect to keep it clean, bacteria can nest in the filter screens, sometimes reaching levels which can make the water from the faucet a problem.

In addition, chlorine may not touch viruses in the water, nor can it eliminate microscopic particles or fibers, such as asbestos, which can pass through various filters. Finally, chlorinating the water does nothing to eliminate industrial pollutants which may be carcinogenic.

Never drink from the hot-water tap. When water is heated, its oxygen bubbles to the surface and some escapes. Without this oxygen, the water tastes stale and flat, which is why good cooks never make tea or coffee from reheated water. The water from the hot-water tap in your faucet is constantly heated so that it will be hot when you turn the tap on. As a result, it has lost some of its oxygen and won't taste "fresh" if you drink it. Other than that, though, there is no reason at all not to drink it if you want to; medically and/or nutritionally speaking, it is exactly the same as the water from the cold tap.

Always let the water run from the tap awhile before you drink it. First of all, it will taste better, since running the cold-water tap chills and aerates it. More important, it may turn out to be better for your health to let the water run a while before you drink it. Especially if your water is *soft*.

Hard water is called "hard" because it contains a lot of minerals, notably calcium and magnesium. These minerals may leave a scum on your hair or clothes, but they also coat the pipes through which the water travels, laying down a protective skim so that the metals in the pipes rarely leach out into the water. Soft water, on the other hand, contains little calcium or magnesium. It is acidic and may dissolve metals such as cadmium, lead, or copper out of the pipes through which it goes. Letting the water run for a few minutes means that you won't get a mouthful of the metal-laden water which has been collecting in the turned-off tap; the running water will still contain metals, but less of them.

For the record, you may wish to know that the hardest water comes from underground wells in the West and Midwest; the softest, or most acidic, from the surface reservoirs of the East and Northeast.

Never drink from the bathroom tap. When the bathroom was first moved indoors and drainage systems were primitive, there is no doubt that the possibility existed that sewage could mix with the tap water. However, in a well-maintained modern bathroom, there is no intermingling of the two, and you can drink at will from any tap you wish. The fact that the same people who think it's dangerous to drink from the bathroom taps brush their teeth in the water there only serves to illustrate the occasionally stunning perversity of the human mind.

Bottled water is better for you than tap water. It depends on what's in the bottle. If the bottled water is truly mineral water, which has a higher mineral content and less sodium than purified and softened tap water, then it may be a better bargain, nutritionally speaking. On the other hand, you have to be careful about what you buy. Bottled water isn't strictly regulated and you may end up buying bottled tap water. And, if the company which bottles the water doesn't pay close attention to its hygiene, the water in the bottle may be teeming with bacteria.

To get the most for your money (and it may be a hefty sum of money—some bottled waters sell for more than a dollar a quart), follow a few common-sense rules: (1) Check the bottle cap to be sure it is sealed tight so that there has been no substitution of contents and so that no air could get in to contaminate the water. (2) Watch out for imprecise label terms. The words "spring fresh" don't mean a thing, and your best bet is sticking to waters from well-known spas either in this country or in Europe.

weather.

It's not the heat, it's the humidity. Actually, it's neither one. The real culprit is the air pressure, which, in hot and humid weather, is generally lower than normal. This lowered pressure of the air against your body allows your tissues to soak up available moisture from the atmosphere and, on a hot and humid day, there's a lot of moisture around to soak up. As the moisture moves into your tissues, you may think of yourself as feeling waterlogged, which, in a way, you are. All that extra moisture can make you feel heavier and slower, and it can even affect your thinking processes. Your skull is hard bone and cannot expand. So, as the tissues of the brain absorb moisture, like all the other tissues in your body, the veins and arteries inside the skull are compressed. That means that the blood flows more slowly through your brain and the supply of oxygen to the brain slows too. The result is dulled thinking, which quickens only when you get into a less moist environment, either inside an air-conditioned room or outside, when the weather changes.

wet feet.

If your feet get wet, you'll get a cold. For more than thirty years, researchers at various universities around this country have been trying to give people colds by dunking them, feet first, into cold water. Unless the cold water was in a room with some active cold viruses, however, nobody ever got a cold that way.

willow bark.

Willow-bark tea cures fevers and pain. The willow tree, whose Latin family name is *Salicaceae,* is rich in salicin, a naturally occurring relative of the laboratory-synthesized medicine which we know as acetylsalicylic acid, or aspirin. Simply chewing the tree's leaves or bark was often as effective as drinking a tea brewed from them, and the willow tree was a staple of folk medicine as far back as the Romans, and probably beyond them, too.

Salicylates first came to the attention of organized medicine late in the eighteenth century. The fashion of the medical day then was an idea called "the doctrine of signatures," which said, simply, that wherever there was a disease, nature had provided a remedy. The point was that you had to look for it. In a paper delivered to the Royal Society of England in 1763, the Reverend Edward Stone allowed as how he had found the cure for the aches and pains associated with moist, damp climates in a tree which flourished in moist, damp areas. His tree was the willow, and by the nineteenth century it had been appropriated by science.

The value of the salicylates was first demonstrated around 1850, but the medicine was shelved because it produced miserable side effects, including nausea. By the 1890s, acetylsalicylic acid, much less irritating than the simpler salicylates, had been produced. Aspirin powders became available in small quantities by the turn of the century. Not, however, in quantities sufficient to deal with the first epidemic in which aspirin might have been of major consequence. The flu pandemic of 1918 simply came too soon, and one can only speculate as to the effect an adequate supply of aspirin might have had on the course of the disease. The debilitating fever of the flu was its worst effect and aspirin, of course, relieves a fever.

wine.

Red wine "strengthens" your blood. At first blush, this looks like another example of sympathetic medicine, which says that things which look alike will interact within the body. Red wine looks like blood, ergo, it will have some effect on your blood if you drink it. (The wine, not the blood.)

In scientific truth, however, this may have something to it, so long as what we are talking about is a sweet red wine. Or, for that matter, a sweet white wine. It's the sweetness, not the color that does the trick, because sweet wines have an abundance of fruit sugar in them, and fruit sugar can "bind" the iron in your steak or other foods so that it is more readily absorbed by your body. No wine can do that on its own, of course, without food, because there is no appreciable amount of iron (the *real* blood "strengthener") in the wine. (NOTE: Pregnant women should never use wine—or any other alcoholic beverage—as a "tonic." Recent research seems to indicate that even 3 ounces of alcohol a day may be injurious to the fetus.)

Drinking wine can protect you against germs. Both wine and grape juice can inactivate bacteria and viruses *in vitro* (in a test tube), as demonstrated in experiments performed in 1977 by two researchers at Health and Welfare Canada. The anti-bacterial and anti-viral effects of the beverages, however, is limited and studies supported by the Concord Grape Association and Welch Foods show that the inactivated organisms come to life again once they are removed from test tubes and exposed to living hosts. Just about the only value they have to us as anti-germ potions is if they are spilled on open wounds, as washes to prevent infection.

work.

Hard work never hurt anyone. It depends on what you mean by "hard work." If you mean continuing physical effort, there is a lot of evidence that hard work—providing, of course, that you get an adequate diet and adequate rest when you're not working—can be a positive boon. In one pioneering study, two researchers at the University of California School of Public Health followed six thousand men for more than ten years. They found that only half as many men who did heavy physical work right up to the days of their deaths tended to die from heart disease as did men who engaged in light or moderate work.

Men (and, increasingly, women) who think that hard work means constantly frustrating situations with little or no opportunity for the release of physical or emotional tension, however, do not profit from their toil. In fact, they show the stress in all the diseases of a civilized world: heart attacks, ulcers, migraine headaches, and the like.

wrinkles.

Staying in water too long will make your hands and feet wrinkle up like prunes. True. There are no sebaceous glands on your palms or on the soles of your feet. The sebaceous glands are the ones which secrete the sticky, fatty lubricant called sebum. Without at least a nominal coating of sebum to repel water, the skin absorbs the water, swells and begins to wrinkle.

See also FACE/FACIAL EXPRESSION.

X

⁜

x-ray.

Dental X-rays are harmless. They may not be. Radiation from X-ray machines is measured in terms of rad or millirads, terms which describe Radiation Absorbed Dosage, or the actual amount of ionizing radiation which penetrates your body during any one X-ray procedure. (There are 1,000 millirads in a rad.)

The newest, most efficient and safest dental X-ray machines deliver about 2 millirads of radiation per picture. But there are still some machines in use which can deliver up to 10 millirads per picture. That means that a set of 20 dental X-rays could give you anywhere from 40 to 200 millirads of radiation. (For purposes of comparison, you get about 200 millirads from one chest X-ray, taken with a good modern machine.)

All X-rays, or ionizing radiation, destroy some body cells. If you get a really massive dose, the destruction can be devastating enough to cause death immediately. A dose of 450 to 600 rads, for example, will be instantly fatal for 50 percent of the people exposed to it. The rest of the people exposed to it will most likely develop cancers such as leukemia from which they die later on.

Nobody yet knows how many cells are damaged by very small doses of radiation, or how long it takes the body to repair and replace the cells, if indeed they can be repaired or replaced at all. In addition, the damage from ionizing radiation is cumulative, which means that serious harm may result from multiple exposure to small doses of radiation previously thought to be safe.

For example, we all get about 0.1 rads of radiation each year (100 millirads) simply by living on a planet which is bombarded by radiation from space. Adding to that, even in small amounts, can trigger trouble.

According to research compiled by Alice Stewart and George Kneale of the University of Birmingham in England and Thomas F. Mancuso of the University of Pittsburgh, accumulated exposure to 3.6 rads (3,600 millirads) can double the chances of contracting bone-marrow cancer. Exposure to 13 rads doubles the possibility of lung cancer; 19 rads doubles the rate of cancers of the pancreas, stomach, and large intestines.

In short, *all* X-rays, no matter how "minor," are potentially dangerous, which is why they should be used only when absolutely necessary for diagnosis and treatment, never simply because the patient or the dentist expects them.

Television sets give off dangerous amounts of radiation. There is no question that television sets produced before 1970, when the federal standards on X-ray emission from TV sets went into effect, gave off more radiation than do modern sets. (If your set conforms to the 1970 standards, there will be a notice to that effect on a sticker or label on the back of the set.)

Whether or not modern TVs give off more radiation than is good for you is a toss-up. People who believe that the only permissible radiation leakage is no radiation leakage will find the TV set dangerous, since if you sit right up close to it (about eight inches away), you are sitting in front of a machine which gives off about 0.5 milliroentgen (pronounce: milly-runt-gen) an hour. A milliroentgen is a unit of radiation which is given off by a source of radiation. To give you an idea of how your television set compares to, say, a dental X-ray machine, it is possible to simply equate a milliroentgen with a millirad. That means that if your dental X-ray machine is a really efficient one, giving you about 2 millirads for each X-ray picture and 40 millirads for a 20-picture series, you would have to sit with your nose pressed against the set for more than 80 hours to get the same amount of radiation from the set as from the X-rays. And remember, as soon as you move more than 8 inches away from the set, the amount of radiation reaching you drops off precipitously to practically nothing.

As of now, HEW considers that a reasonable risk to take. Whether or not it will seem as reasonable ten or twenty years from now is anyone's guess, since the level of officially acceptable radiation exposure continues to drop as we learn more about the true amounts necessary to trigger injuries within the human body.

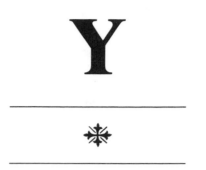

Y

yogurt.

Eating yogurt cures vaginitis. Sometimes women who use antibiotics find that the medication destroys the lactobacilli, or good bacteria, in the vaginal area, allowing other bacteria or yeasts to proliferate. The result is a vaginal infection caused by micro-organism imbalance.

Since some yogurts contain live lactobacilli*, many women assume that by eating yogurt they can replenish the bacterial supply in the vaginal area and avoid or cure the infection. However, the lactobacilli taken by mouth will not reach the vaginal area alive, since the acid condition of the stomach is quite inhospitable for them. Applying yogurt to the vaginal area will put the bacteria where they are needed, but it is a messy procedure and, if the yogurt is not removed, it will simply rot there.

It makes more sense, both medically and aesthetically, to douche with warm water in which you have put some plain yogurt culture (the bacteria, without the milk). But one must always be certain that

---

*The bacteria in a yogurt such as Light 'n Lively which is "ultrapasteurized," pasteurized *after* culturing, are dead, or at least not plentiful enough to be of any medical value.

the treatment is called for. A lot of things, including venereal disease, can look like a simple vaginitis, and yogurt or yogurt culture will do them no good at all, and may even do harm by keeping you away from necessary medical treatment.

Yogurt cures constipation. Although all milk products can cause constipation from time to time, there has been some evidence that yogurt works the other way, relieving constipation in geriatric patients. The study most often cited involved 194 senior citizens at a New York hospital. Their constipation responded favorable to daily helpings of yogurt. However, the yogurt used in the study was prune-whip yogurt, which may raise some questions as to which of the ingredients was doing the real work.

Yogurt cures diarrhea. Yogurt has been shown to be more effective than ordinary antibiotics in curing infant diarrhea. In 1963, there was a report in *Clinical Pediatrics,* a medical journal, detailing the results of a study done at the Department of Pediatrics at Jewish Memorial Hospital in New York, in which one group of sick infants were given neomycin and another yogurt. The babies on yogurt did better than those on neomycin, and, several years later, in another study, yogurt alone also outperformed a combination of neomycin and Kaopectate. There have been no comparative studies done on adults with diarrhea.

Eating yogurt before you go abroad can prevent turista. The assumption is that you will build up a supply of good bacteria to knock off the bad. It has never been proven, one way or the other.

Yogurt cures a sunburn. It is a cool, wet dressing, which can make the burned area feel better, but like butter on a burn, yogurt on a sunburn can create a layer of food over an injured area and may possibly lead to an infection if it is not removed.

Z

❋

---

zinc oxide.

Zinc oxide ointment keeps your nose from getting sunburned. Absolutely. The thick, white ointment is actually a physical barrier which prevents the sun's burning rays from getting through to your skin. The only drawback, of course, is precisely that the stuff is thick and white—it looks awful. Which is why thin lotions with a chemical sunscreen such as PABA are so much more popular for whole-body protection.

Index

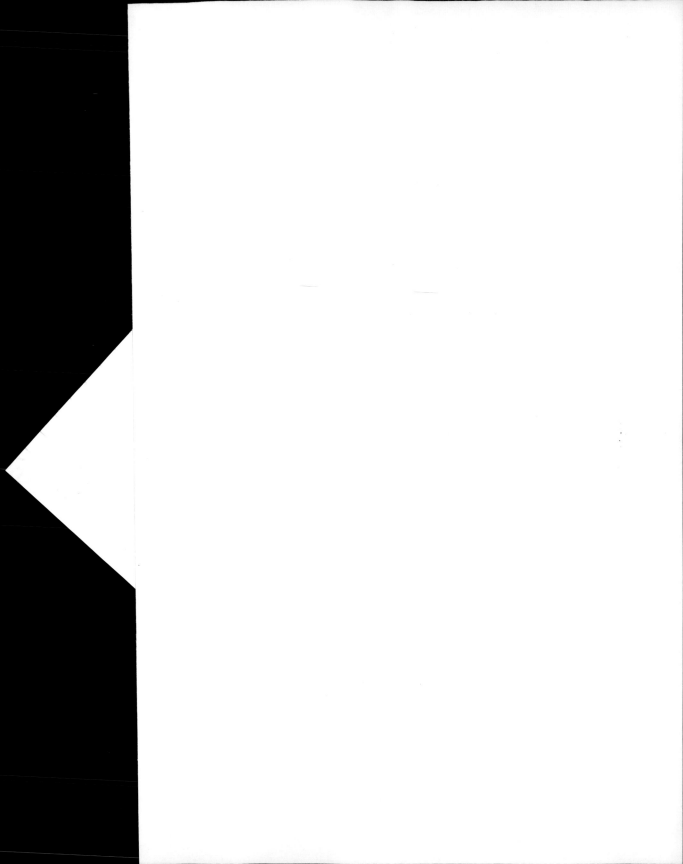